"This thoughtful, well-written, insightful best book available for couples who want understand why sexual desire decreases and, based on this understanding, learn how to increase sensual/sexual desires, passion, and emotional closeness. *In the Mood, Again* will help couples fight for their marriage and restore, protect, and ensure a lasting love based on friendship, knowledge, and desire."

> —Howard J. Markman, Ph.D., professor of psychology, director of the Center for Marital and Family Studies at the University of Denver and coauthor, *We Can Work It Out* and *Fighting for Your Marriage*

"This book is a must-have for every practitioner of women's health care. In clear and concise language, Cervenka unravels the mystery of sexuality and provides practical substantiated advice that will improve the quality of life for women of all ages. It is a treasure of valuable and useful clinical information."

> —Mary Lee Josey, MD, Diplomate, American Board of Obstetrics and Gynecology, fellow, American College of Obstetrics and Gynecology

"From a sex expert who tells it like it is, comes the skinny on what really works to recharge a couple's sex life. Cervenka knows it's not about blaming one or another partner, but helping both partners tap into their sexual power and communicate in ways that will turn up the heat. This is a fun and important book."

> —Lauren Dockett, coauthor of *Sex Talk* and author of *The Deepest Blue*

"Finally, a book that deals honestly and candidly with many issues and insecurities that couples in mature relationships often do not know how to approach. For women in long-lasting relationships who feel that sex is just one more chore, this book is your lifeline! Throughout this delightful, often witty and utterly truthful book Cervenka presents couples with concrete examples and practical exercises that will help re-ignite the flame you thought was lost forever. I highly recommend this book to anyone who has lost desire for their partner and wishes to invest in this most important relationship."

—Amy Borenstein, Ph.D., MPH, professor, College of Public Health, University of South Florida

"This is a book for couples of all ages. Filled with insights gained from years of experience as a sex therapist, this guide focuses on the importance of desire, the largely unappreciated antecedent to an enduring emotional and sexual relationship. Seniors need to hear more about enduring love and sexual desire and less about the declining frequency of sexual activity with increasing age. I highly recommend this book to them."

—James A. Mortimer, Ph.D., Saunders professor of Gerontology and director of the Institute on Aging at the University of South Florida

In the *Mood,* Again

A Couple's Guide to Reawakening Sexual Desire

Kathleen A. Cervenka, Ph.D.

New Harbinger Publications, Inc.

Publisher's Note

This publication is designed to provide accurate and authoritative information in regard to the subject matter covered. It is sold with the understanding that the publisher is not engaged in rendering psychological, financial, legal, or other professional services. If expert assistance or counseling is needed, the services of a competent professional should be sought.

Distributed in the U.S.A. by Publishers Group West; in Canada by Raincoast Books; in Great Britain by Hi Marketing, Ltd.; in South Africa by Real Books, Ltd.; in Australia by Boobook; and in New Zealand by Tandem Press.

Copyright © 2003 by Kathleen Cervenka
New Harbinger Publications, Inc.
5674 Shattuck Avenue
Oakland, CA 94609

Cover design by Amy Shoup
Cover image by J.P. Nacivet/Getty Images
Text design by Michele Waters

ISBN 1-57224-351-1 Paperback

Printed in the United States of America

New Harbinger Publications' Web site address: www.newharbinger.com

05   04   03

10 9 8 7 6 5 4 3 2 1

First printing

This book is dedicated with everything I am, with all my spirit, and with my deepest, eternal love to my magnificent husband, Hendricks, whose gentle and loving spirit epitomizes the definition of a passionate relationship.

To my children, Chris and Joe, whose brilliance, sensitivity, and humor continue to inspire me. And to Jim, who is a loving addition to our family.

Contents

Acknowledgments

My deepest gratitude goes to my loving husband, Hendricks, for his endless patience, intuitive insight, brilliant guidance, and constant encouragement offered throughout this venture. The completion of this book would not have been possible without his empowerment. The love and passion experienced in our relationship epitomizes what I wish for all couples reading this book.

I thank my glorious daughter, Chris, for making me laugh hard when I felt my power diminishing. Her humor, intelligence, and generous heart encouraged me to tap into my power. She and her wonderful husband, Jim, offered countless hours of feedback throughout the various versions of this book, thus ensuring that joy, love, and humor were present throughout each chapter.

I thank my magnificent son, Joe, for his perceptiveness in knowing exactly when and how to empower me during this arduous task. He continued to remind me of why I decided to write this book. I am in constant awe of his courage, intelligence, humor, and sensitive nature. Power reciprocity was constant while I discussed this book with him.

Although my parents are deceased, they deserve my heartfelt gratitude for providing me with an outrageously happy upbringing filled with love, laughter, and an atmosphere conducive to building self-confidence. Their spirits cheered me on throughout this process. My siblings, Carol, Joe, Mary, Nancy, and Patty, deserve my thanks for their support as well.

My deepest gratitude goes to Jueli Gastwirth, senior acquisitions editor of New Harbinger Publications, whose vision and dedication made the publication of this book possible. Every person that I had the good fortune to work with at New Harbinger has been warm, accessible, and bright. Thanks to you all: Wendy Millstine, Heather Mitchener, Gretchen Gold, Michele Waters, Lorna Garano, and Amy Shoup.

My heartfelt thanks go out to the hundreds of patients who honored me by their trust, courage, and hard work. It was they who encouraged me to write a book so millions of others could benefit from my approach.

Of course, I could not have written this book without the influence of those brilliant minds that continue to shape the manner in which I provide treatment to couples: Drs. Aaron T. Beck, Salvador Minuchin, Gregory Bateson, Helen Singer Kaplan, William Masters, Virginia Johnson, John Gottman, and Deborah Tannen. A special thank-you goes to Dr. Bill Granzig for being my champion and mentor. Many more of these great minds are listed in the reference section of this book.

My graduate work at the University of Chicago continues to be an ongoing influence in my ability to keep up on current research and prevention studies, which I incorporate throughout my clinical work. My deepest gratitude goes to all the brilliant individuals who comprise this magnificent university.

Discussing sexual issues in the media continues to present controversy from antisexual groups, despite its importance in people's lives. Kathy Fountain, who hosts *Your Turn,* and producer Cindy Simmons courageously aired programs containing sexual content. My deepest gratitude to you both for treating sexual topics with complete respect and dignity.

While attending Roosevelt University from 1976 to 1979, an inspiring female Professor, Marjorie Mayo, became my mentor and friend. Wherever you are, Professor Mayo, I want you to know that you continue to have a powerful influence. Thank you for being a part of my heart and my life.

I am blessed to have great friends that continued to encourage me during the several drafts of my book. To my fellow authors and eloquent writers Laurie Viera and Kathy Baker, for their invaluable input. To Alan, Tonya, Sandy, Jean, and Angela, for being my champions.

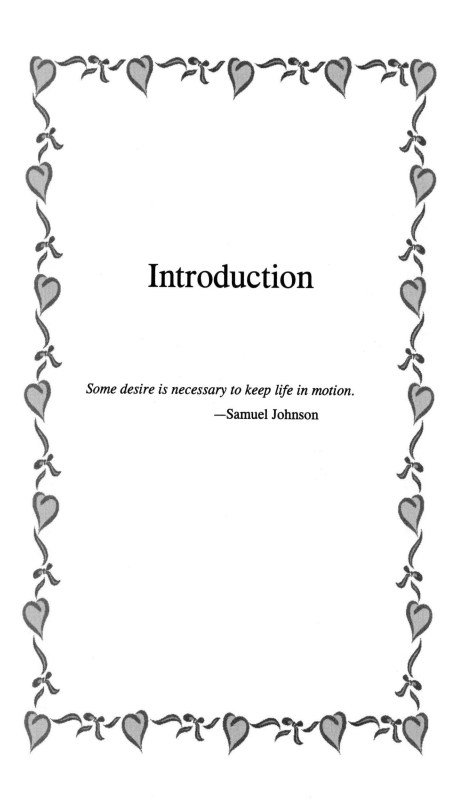

Introduction

Some desire is necessary to keep life in motion.
—Samuel Johnson

Has that flame of passion, once enjoyed between you and your partner, burned out? Has your sex drive dropped drastically compared to what it was in the past? Do you blame your partner? Or, perhaps you blame yourself. Are you wondering why, after months or years of having great sex, the magic is gone? Are you concerned that your sexual desire—or that of your partner—is gone forever? Would you or your partner rather get some sleep, read a book, eat an apple, or talk to your mother-in-law than have sex? If you answered "yes" to any or all of these questions, you and your partner will benefit from this book.

According to most sex therapists, the number of couples requesting treatment for low sexual desire continues to increase. None of us are alone with this problem. In fact, almost all couples will experience a decline in lust at some point in their relationship. The first thing you should notice is that you and your partner are in the company of millions.

You should also know that low sexual desire does not discriminate in terms of gender, race, age, marital status, or sexual orientation. It can hit anyone at anytime. If you are in a loving relationship and you happen to be young or old, gay or straight, married or single, male or female, black, white, green, or purple, you and your partner will come away with a greater understanding from reading this book.

What amazes me when discussing relationships and how to improve our sex lives is that we often treat sexuality as a separate issue. People want to fix their sex lives without dealing with fundamental issues within any intimate relationship. But sexuality cannot be treated as a separate issue. After all, if two mature people love one another, the natural outcome of their love is expressed sexually. With this in mind, I will be discussing love and sex in the same conversation. And inside this conversation live passion and desire—the missing elements that connect us to more satisfying sexual lives.

I know what you're thinking right now. No doubt you thought this book would teach you more creative sexual techniques, like how to have five thousand orgasms, or how to stay erect for over a minute, or how to wrap yourself in plastic wrap, or how to be more romantic by throwing rose petals all over the bed. Instead, our conversation begins with that sensual and lustful feeling that overtook you when you and your partner began to date. You remember those days. This book is designed to help you get those passionate feelings back! Of course, I'm not implying that you shouldn't experiment with novel sexual techniques. You can, but if sexual desire is missing, these techniques will be like drinking a warm, flat glass of champagne: no bubbles, no zip, and little taste. You are free to drink flat champagne if you choose. However, if you're like most, you prefer your champagne chilled and bubbly.

I'm certain that most of you had no idea that your relationship was suffering from what clinicians call a sexual desire disorder. When there is an interference with the natural sexual motivation system, this is called hypoactive sexual desire disorder (HSD). Some of you will feel distressed and others will feel relief that there is actually a name for what you have. Either way, I want you both to feel the excitement in knowing that there is something you can do to ameliorate this disorder. The passion once experienced during the initial phase of your relationship is just waiting to be reawakened. You will soon discover this for yourselves, once I take you and your partner through this exhilarating process.

I have worked with hundreds of couples just like you who suffered greatly when one member of the relationship is no longer interested in any type of sexual activity, but the other is. After all, sex is an extremely important component of any loving relationship. The discovery that a desire disorder is temporary should offer you and your partner a great deal of relief. Recapturing desire, however, requires work by both you and your partner.

As mentioned, over the past twenty-three years, I have treated hundreds of couples in my private practice who have suffered from low or nonexistent sexual desire. As a cognitive/systems therapist, as well as a human sexuality clinician, I approach the issue of low or nonexistent sexual desire as a couple, rather than an individual, issue. That means I will be talking to both of you throughout this book. At its core, low sexual desire is a relationship issue; its solution will involve both of you.

Besides my work in private practice, I often appear on television and the radio. While I discuss a wide range of topics addressing relationships and family issues in the media, there is absolutely nothing that generates as much intense interest as low sexual desire. I sometimes get the impression that, at some point in time, everyone on this planet experiences a drop in libido. Although it is extremely common, it is frightening when it happens to you. Media is a great vehicle for raising awareness about sexual desire. It does not, however, provide the time, nor the intimacy, needed to have an impact on couples. Only by writing a book could I share my clinical experience with as many people as possible.

While writing this book, I felt I knew you personally. How, you ask? At our cores, we are all human beings with similar needs. You want to be understood, accepted, loved, and honored for exactly who you are. You want to feel connected to that one special person with whom you chose to share your life.

I am fortunate enough to be sharing my life with an incredibly awesome man who is the love of my life. Our twenty-three-year relationship has brought much happiness, peace, joy, and passion. All of these feelings, as you will soon discover, live inside of individual power and power reciprocity, and this power is manifest through connected conversations.

My wish is for everyone to experience the rewards of an empowered sexual relationship. I know you love each other, but you've experienced sexual frustration and disappointment in your relationship. Welcome to the real world. No, love doesn't conquer all, but possessing individual power and power reciprocity does. Simply stated, individual power is the ability to be influential, convincing, and persuasive, and having the capacity of producing a positive effect on your partner. Power reciprocity is the ability to empower your partner and to allow your partner to empower you as well. But how on earth are you supposed to have an empowering relationship if you haven't been taught? You cannot learn how to speak Czechoslovakian if someone doesn't teach you the basics of the language. Once you learn the basics, you then have the choice of learning enough to get by or becoming fluent. Yet, most of us believe that we can enter a relationship without learning the basics. There is no such thing as winging it.

In spite of everything that is universally true about all of us, I understand that every relationship is unique. Yes, we all have similar needs. However, these needs are expressed in unique ways within each individual relationship. For this reason, I will be presenting you with lots of different ideas to help you improve the quality of your sexually loving relationship. Some of them will fit and others will not. Focus on the ideas that fit and practice using them without delay.

I realize that there can be painful feelings attached to what I'm asking you to do; if your sex life were perfect or you had no concerns about the future, you would not have bought this book. But the benefits of this book to your life are pretty obvious and valuable—a powerful, intimate, connected relationship and more passionate sex. Having power and returning it to your partner result in a sizzling sex life. Actually, there are few relationships that do not need sexual improvement. At least you have the courage to reach out and admit that your sex life needs improvement, and you are willing to do something about it. Bravo for you!

I have some requests that I would like you to follow. Please do not jump around in the book. I understand how it feels to want to get to the essence of a book; however, I want you to resist the temptation. Every chapter builds on the previous one. If you skip a chapter, you will interrupt the momentum of this process. Remember, this is the exact process that I take my clients through in couple therapy. Take each chapter as it comes, and I promise you will reap the benefits. Keep in mind that you are saving thousands of therapeutic dollars. That should be an incentive!

Throughout the book, I will ask you to engage in various exercises. Make sure you have pen and paper for these exercises. Please do each and every exercise. I will coach you both through each one. They are not meant to embarrass you or your partner. They're meant to be used as a guideline to indicate where you and your partner are regarding the particular issue that we are exploring. Sometimes one person is more eager to engage in exercises than the other is. However, if you both don't do all of these exercises, I cannot guarantee that you will have the same results my clients successfully experience in my private practice.

Finally, I must request that you and your partner give up, or at least set aside, your guilt and shame when it comes to discussing sexual issues. I will be discussing graphic sexual issues throughout this book. I appreciate fully that sexuality is a private matter that demands the utmost respect. It is not my wish to shock or embarrass you. This is an intimate book that was written in the spirit of love and respect for you and your partner to explore privately. Hopefully, by the end of this book, you will feel comfortable discussing sexual issues with your partner without shame or embarrassment.

The whole idea of reading this book is to create an opening for you and your partner to become powerful, to have power reciprocity in your relationship, and to be able to use this power to engage in connected conversations. This, in turn, will provide you both with an intimate and passionate relationship that is beyond what you have ever dreamed of experiencing!

This book was intentionally designed to be free of any technical language. Clinicians are famous for using complex terminology. Yet, most of us would prefer comprehensive language that is straightforward and authentic. Even without using technical language, this book was written also for clinicians who are seeking to address the sexual concerns of their clients. It is an excellent book to use as an adjunct to therapy. Clinicians should keep in mind that this book addresses only hypoactive desire disorder. It does not address sex aversion or hyperactive sexual desire disorders. As clinicians know, these disorders must be addressed in a professional setting.

Clinicians should also note that I treat HSD as completely separate from the genital phase disorders of arousal and orgasm. As you will most likely recognize, my approach is systemic, cognitively based, and at times, psychoanalytic in nature. Taking a systems point of view, the couple is treated rather than the individual. If you are a clinician, I hope you enjoy the book, and may it enhance the many skills and the knowledge base that you already have.

On a last note: all the case illustrations are disguised in order not to betray any confidentiality agreements. This book, as in most, is not meant as a replacement for professional treatment for more severe sexual problems.

Now, let's get going. Happy reading and have fun!

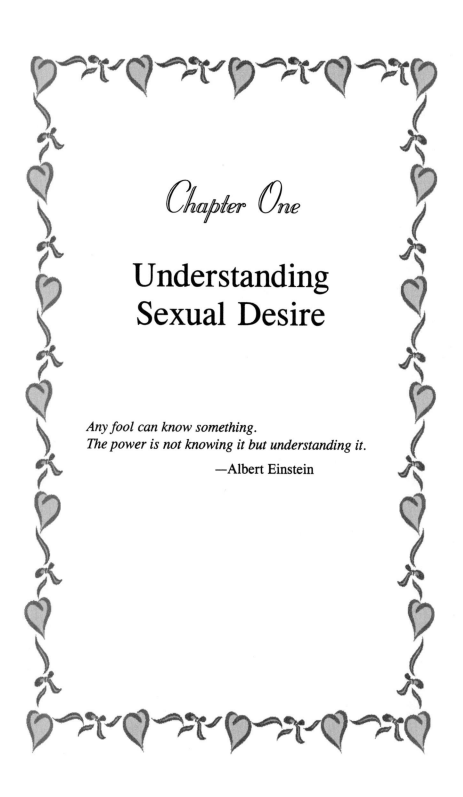

Chapter One

Understanding
Sexual Desire

Any fool can know something.
The power is not knowing it but understanding it.

—Albert Einstein

Millions of men and women, involved in loving relationships, are currently experiencing a lack of sexual desire. I've spent most of my professional career treating these couples. When an individual, once sexually active, loses their desire to engage in sexual activities, we clinicians refer to this condition as hypoactive sexual desire disorder. This condition usually causes a great deal of stress not only on the individual suffering from a desire disorder, but on the relationship as well. Why are so many individuals suffering from this drop in libido? You will soon discover answers to this complex and perplexing problem throughout this chapter.

Typical questions couples ask are, "Why did I look forward to having sex with my partner when we first got together, but now I couldn't care less if I ever have sex again? What happened to our once sexy and intimate relationship? Does this mean that I'm no longer in love with my partner? Does this mean that my partner is no longer attracted to me? Can we ever recapture the lust we once experienced together? Is this a normal occurrence that happens to most couples? Or, are there more serious problems that we need to resolve within our relationship? Should I pretend everything is fine and go through the motions of having sex with my partner, even though I don't feel like it?"

If you or your partner have asked yourselves any of these questions, I'm sure you're concerned that your once cherished relationship is in serious jeopardy. Well, put your worry aside. Almost everyone, at some point in his or her relationship, goes through a drop in libido. In order to begin the process of recapturing sexual desire, it is imperative that you first have a clear understanding of what desire is all about. Sexual desire marks the beginning phases of the Human Sexual Response Cycle (Masters and Johnson 1966). Let's briefly go through these phases together.

The Human Sexual Response Cycle

Masters and Johnson (1966) originally conceptualized this model to explain the distinct and highly pleasurable phases that an individual goes through to prepare oneself for procreation. Helen Singer Kaplan (1974) collapsed their version and created a more succinct one, known as the Tri-Phasic Model. I prefer Kaplan's simpler version.

Phase One: Desire

During this phase our brain's sexual motivational system is the major player. This motivation is what leads us towards a deeply emotional, willful expression of our love for one another.

If something interferes with this motivation, a desire disorder can occur. Disorders within this phase are hypoactive sexual desire disorder (low or absent desire), hyperactive sexual desire disorder (sexual addiction), and sexual aversion (a phobic reaction to a partner). This book focuses only on hypoactive sexual desire disorder, the most prevalent of the desire disorders.

Phase Two: Arousal (Excitement)

During this phase the parasympathetic nervous system is the major player. Any type of sexual stimulation elicits neurological, vascular, muscular, and hormonal reactions affecting the entire body. Genital changes are brought about by vasocongestion (filling with blood). The most significant physical changes in women are the vagina begins to lubricate and the clitoris becomes enlarged. In men, the penis becomes erect and the testicles are drawn up towards the body. For both men and women the nipples may become erect.

Dysfunctions occurring within this phase are male erectile disorder (impotency) and female sexual arousal disorder (inability to lubricate adequately). This phase is not addressed in this book.

Phase Three: Orgasm

During this most pleasurable phase, the sympathetic nervous system is the major player. Increased muscle tension is experienced, and then released throughout the body. Women experience contractions of the uterus and vagina, resulting in a general loss of voluntary muscle control. Men experience contractions in the prostate gland, the urethral bulb, and the tubes that produce and carry sperm from the testes, resulting in ejaculation.

Dysfunctions occurring within this phase are female orgasmic disorder (inability to achieve orgasm following adequate sexual stimulation), male orgasmic disorder (inability to achieve orgasm following adequate sexual stimulation), and premature ejaculation (ejaculating before or very shortly after penile insertion). These are not addressed in this book.

We should note, however, that there are several books explaining the arousal and orgasmic phases, and appropriate treatments for those disorders. Very few books emphasize the desire phase, with the exception of Helen Singer Kaplan's (1995) book for clinicians on the sexual desire disorders.

Why Make a Distinction between the Desire and the Genital Phases?

The answer is simple. If you don't understand the difference between the desire phase and the genital phases, the treatment won't fit the diagnosis. Many, but not all, clinicians begin offering treatment that doesn't fit with a desire disorder. It is crucial that the treatment procedure fits the diagnosis. The treatment, offered within these pages, is specifically designed for couples who simply can't get in the mood.

Sexual Desire Is Motivation

Sexual desire is a motivational system. Motivation works in a similar fashion as the drive to eat or drink. Our brain lets us know when we are hungry or thirsty without much conscious thought. It is the same with sexual motivation. If your frequency of sexual activity is weekly, and you have not had sex for several weeks, you will be more motivated to engage in sexual activities. On the other hand, if you have had sex an hour ago, your drive will likely be low. But what happens when you have not had sex for weeks or even months, and you still do not feel like engaging in any type of sexual activity? It means that something is interfering with your sexual drive centers, and they are temporarily turned off.

What Regulates This Motivational System?

A small portion of your brain, called the hypothalamus, contains these tiny sexual drive centers that are activated by external and internal signals. The late Helen Singer Kalpan (1995) coined the phrase, "sex centers"—I like that, so that's the term I'll use throughout the book. An external signal that would activate your sex centers is when you view your partner as sexually attractive, powerful, and loving. An internal signal is when you view yourself as sexually attractive, powerful, and loving. These signals regulate our sex drive.

What's behind the Sex Drive?

All animals, including human beings, have a sex drive. The fundamental reason for this drive is to keep our species alive through procreation. To reinforce this sex drive, nature made intercourse extremely pleasurable. But we all know that the conscious aim of procreating is not the dominant reason for having sex. There are millions of gays and lesbians, involved in loving relationships, where procreation is impossible (at least with each other directly). These couples certainly do possess a healthy sex drive, because of the intense pleasure sexuality creates. There are also many heterosexual couples who have zero intention of procreating. They may not want children, but they certainly want to experience sexual pleasure. And let's not forget the couples who already have had children and are past their childbearing years. Their sex drive does not disappear simply because the body is no longer able to bear children.

Is Physical Pleasure the Major Force behind the Sex Drive?

For most of us, being sexual means more than experiencing a few fleeting moments (or hours) of pleasure. Most of us need to feel an intimate connection with our partner. Sharing our body involves manifesting our deep love through the most intimate and spiritual connection we can have in our relationship. That's why most of us refer to sexual intercourse as making love. Of course, intercourse is only one out of thousands of ways that we express our love for one another sexually. Any intimate act—such as kissing, touching, speaking to another sexually, or listening to the sexual talk of your partner—is a sexual activity. A more graphic discussion will take place during the last chapter.

Does the Intensity of This Sex Drive Change during One's Lifetime?

Thankfully, it does. During adolescence, our sex drive is at its peak and gradually slows down each year thereafter. That's not to say that our sex drive ever stops completely. There are many studies that prove that the elderly continue to experience a sex drive and enjoy love-making. It is just not as often.

Do All Couples Have the Same Sex Drive?

No, absolutely not. Whatever works for the two of you is considered normal. Do not get so sucked into sexual stories presented on the soaps, talk shows, and movies that entice you to believe that normality must mean everyone has a sex drive that thrusts you into having sex three times a day. Although it is amusing to watch these fantasy couples with voracious sex drives frolicking in the elevator, on top of the kitchen counter, on a public beach, or on an airplane, most people consider these a special treat, not an everyday meal. It's a fantasy, albeit a fun and exciting one. Most of us, however, prefer the comfort of a mattress, in private, using one of our favored positions.

But what about couples who make love as much as three times a day or as little as once a year? Would this be considered *normal?*

Of course it would. Normal is what you and your partner decide is normal. It simply does not matter whether you fall into the high end or the low end of the sex drive spectrum. What is important is that you both feel satisfied with this frequency.

Does Frequency Present Problems?

Frequency is a problem only if one partner desires sex more than their partner. The spectrum of human sexual desire is a broad one, and it is just one of the many things that makes each of us unique. Most of us know what is normal or usual for ourselves in terms of our sex drive.

Those who are generally at the high end of the desire spectrum would consider themselves to be extremely sexual beings. They enjoy enormously the experience of being sexual and in a perfect world would love to have sex daily. The very thought of their partner is enough to make them want to rush home and make love.

Those who are generally at the low end of the desire spectrum also enjoy being sexual, but with less frequency. They simply do not feel the need for sex as often. When they do engage in sex, they experience intense pleasure in expressing their love. And certainly there are a thousand levels of desire between these two ends of the spectrum. It will be up to you and your partner to determine some type of compromise.

How Would the Desire Discrepancy Manifest Itself?

The first scenario is when two people form a relationship and discover that one is on the high end of the desire spectrum and the other is on the low end. Some couples confront this issue early in the relationship; others might grudgingly and resentfully resign themselves to it for many years. This scenario usually represents a basic compatibility issue that can be resolved by compromise.

The second scenario is when both partners have a history of generally being in sync in terms of their desire, and then one partner loses interest in having sex. This scenario is what causes so many problems, and it nearly always points to a lack of individual power and power reciprocity within the relationship.

The third scenario is when one partner has a drop in libido and the other adapts to this drop by developing a desire disorder as well. Usually, when one recaptures his or her desire, the other recaptures desire as well.

Could a Drop in Libido Mean that There Is Something Wrong with You?

Whenever something doesn't *feel right,* you have to explore the recent changes in your life. A drop in libido could signal a physical, pharmacological, emotional, or interpersonal problem. There are also factors like depression, anxiety, stress, or physical maladies that can contribute to having a low libido. Take the time to reflect on your mental, emotional, and physical state in order to understand what's having an impact on your life.

The most common reason, however, is interpersonal. In all my twenty-three years in clinical practice, I have yet to treat individuals who have serious physical problems that cause lack of desire. It is wise, however, to get checked out by a physician just in case. I mostly see couples who have become disenchanted with either themselves or their partners. They don't seem to respond to any type of erotic stimulation. They seldom engage in sexual fantasy. Nor do they have the urge to masturbate. In other words, if their partner jumped out of a cake buck naked, their response would be, "Well, that was entertaining, but no thanks." Even if they try, they find it extremely difficult getting their sex centers turned on. If, however, their partner successfully talks them into having sex, they could possibly enjoy the sexual experience. There is no question, however, that when sexual desire is present rather than coaxed, the enjoyment is highly intensified.

Does Testosterone Increase Sexual Desire?

Yes, if your sex drive is depleted because your testosterone level is below normal. A popular notion, directed towards women, is if she slathers on some ointment, pops a pill, plasters on a patch, or takes an injection, this additional testosterone can turn her into a sex goddess. The truth is, if a woman has too much of this hormone, she'll turn into the antithesis of a sex goddess. Be forewarned; never consider taking testosterone supplements without consulting a physician first. Too much testosterone in a woman can cause masculine side effects such as hair loss, acne, increased facial hair growth, loss of breast fat, and a deepened voice. This has actually happened to some women who decided that supplementing their body's natural production of testosterone would increase their sexual desire. They read somewhere that testosterone increased desire and decided to take this hormone without a physician's exam or a hormone check. When they began to develop these side effects, they immediately discontinued use and the side effects disappeared, with the exception of the deepened voice. Once a voice deepens, it will never be restored back to normal; that's permanent damage.

A person's own testosterone level is the key to their sexual desire. The androgen testosterone is, in fact, responsible for turning on the receptors of our sex centers. Actually, testosterone is usually referred to as the "libido or desire hormone."

Many of us think of testosterone as an exclusively male hormone. This, however, is a misnomer. Women produce testosterone as well. In males, it is primarily produced in the testicles; in females, it is produced in the ovaries. To a lesser extent, the adrenal glands of both men and women also manufacture testosterone. Testosterone is critical and accountable for both male and female sex drives. You must maintain adequate levels to have a healthy sexual desire.

Even though it is a minimal probability that a woman's testosterone level will be too low, all women should have their testosterone levels checked by a gynecologist, particularly if they have had a total hysterectomy (removal of the uterus and ovaries) or are beginning menopause. Here is why this is so important. If the ovaries were removed along with the uterus, or the ovaries have run out of eggs, testosterone is no longer released from that site. It is possible that you would then not produce enough testosterone. However, most women do not have to worry about this, because the adrenal glands will continue to secrete testosterone and compensate for what the ovaries used to produce.

Similarly, it is highly unusual for adult males to have an abnormally low level of testosterone. Even if the male's testes have been injured or removed because of an illness, the adrenal glands will generally compensate for the loss. Nonetheless, if you suspect that for some reason your testosterone levels are below normal, have a doctor check your levels. If your doctor then concludes that your levels are low, taking supplemental testosterone under a doctor's supervision can possibly raise your level of sexual desire.

The Five Sensations of Desire

The most common motivators to sexual desire include anything and everything that your mind perceives as erotic. These erotic sensations are stimulated by touching, seeing, smelling, tasting, and hearing. To heighten these erotic sensations is the ability to engage in sexual fantasy. Let's take a brief look at what can turn on those sex centers.

Touch

Many individuals state that a touch behind the ear, behind the knee, the inner thigh, the palm of the hand, the neck, the back, the buttocks, the toes, the feet, the breasts, the stomach, or any place else you can think of, can elicit intense sexual desire. Our skin offers sexual pleasure because there are nerve endings that send a signal to the brain that something really great is happening. This touch can turn on those sex centers in the brain and signal pure lust. However, this touch has to be perceived as something pleasurable, based on the circumstances of the touch. For example, if you're on the subway and the stranger next to you places his hand on your knee, chances are you'll have a major creep attack and your sex centers will be turned off. But if you are in a darkened movie theater and your partner touches your knee, you will experience erotic pleasure.

Smell

Another sense that elicits sexual desire is the olfactory. You may love the smell of your partner's genitals, which can lead to desire. Or you may be repulsed by the odor, which will cause those sex centers to slam shut. Olfactory eroticism is totally subjective.

A sensory turn-on can change due to circumstances, and the sense of smell is a particularly evocative one. Let's say that your partner brings home your favorite flowers that you've always loved for their smell. Usually, you would experience sensual pleasure. However, let's say that a close friend has recently passed away, and the smell now reminds you of the funeral home. This sense memory fills you with sadness, and your sex centers are turned off. Your perception of the smell changed drastically based on the circumstances.

It would be impossible to talk about the sense of smell without briefly mentioning pheromones, which have received a lot of media attention in recent years. Pheromones are sex hormones that are released through the skin of both men and women. In the animal kingdom, a female who is in heat secretes these chemicals, which attracts the male and increases his desire to mate. Remember musk oil and perfumes that contained pheromones? Supposedly humans attract one another by secreting similar chemicals, which when inhaled give one a feeling of euphoria and calmness. Although the research conducted in this area is inconclusive regarding sexual desire, many of my patients have told me that they love the natural smell of their partner, which does in fact increase their sexual desire.

Sight

Most of us feel that we are partnered with an attractive person, but again, attraction is totally subjective. What is attractive to one person may be unattractive to another. Nonetheless, we initially choose our partner based on physical attraction. It is only after feeling this initial physical attraction that we get to know our partner's inner qualities.

Nonetheless, there are times that the sight of our otherwise attractive lover can turn us off. Let's say you're in the bedroom feeling quite romantic and your partner comes to bed. The first thing you notice is that he is wearing a ripped T-shirt that is easily three sizes too small. Suddenly you find yourself saying, "Have a nice sleep, see you in the morning." Or your partner comes home early from work hoping to have a romantic moment and finds you wearing a facial mudpack. What happens? He suddenly says, "I'll be back in a couple of hours; I'm going out to play tennis with Bob." Whether we like to admit it or not, an attractive partner is one of the keys to sexual desire.

Hopefully, most of us are not tricked by the fashion and cosmetic industries' version of attractiveness. They create a multibillion-dollar industry based on an illusion of the unattainable. Women watch a slick commercial of another woman applying the lipstick shade of the hour, which transforms her into a luscious femme fatale. The scene has been carefully choreographed, using perfect lighting and a camera lens that erases every imperfection. If the commercial is successful, the woman who watched it runs down to her nearest drugstore and buys that lipstick. Guess what? She's not going to be magically transformed into that illusion of a woman.

Men are far from immune to such messages, both in terms of how they view women and how they view themselves. A man with thinning hair might watch a commercial in which a male actor is as bald as a bowling ball, looking distressed and alone. The lighting is harsh, and the camera lens shows every imperfection imaginable. However, after he applies a solution to his scalp, he now has a full head of hair, the lighting is changed and that magic camera lens is in place. Plus, he's in the company of that lipstick woman running her fingers through his newly grown hair. If the commercial is successful, the men watching that commercial run out to buy that product. Sadly, they are not going to be magically transformed into that male model, nor is lipstick lady going to jump out of the closet.

Attractiveness is based on your unique perception. My partner thinks I'm attractive and vice versa. However, I suppose there are hundreds of others who would disagree with our perceptions. Whose perception counts? What is important is that you perceive yourself and your partner as attractive, not that you conform to the images of perfection that the media would have you believe are the only standard of beauty.

Sound

People are often turned on by listening to music. Let's say that, during that initial phase of your relationship, you were listening to a piece of music and, at the same time, you were making mad, passionate love. Years later, you hear that same piece and you get turned on. Why, you ask? The sound triggered that old feeling of uninhibited lovemaking. Some couples have certain music that they play while making love because it increases sexual desire. Some love the sound of the ocean waves.

Then there are various sounds that can instantly turn off those sex centers, like listening to someone chew with their mouth open or blowing their nose. These sounds would instantly put the brakes on most people's sexual desire.

While individual tastes in sounds vary, most partners love the sound of each other's voices. Remember a time when you and your partner were apart? You picked up the phone and heard your lover's voice. The sound of that voice turned on your sexual desire.

Taste

A sumptuous meal can be a real turn-on. It can be oysters, strawberries, whipped cream, or whatever just happens to be your idea of erotic food. It becomes especially exciting when you eat your favorite treats in bed while in the process of lovemaking. Some couples love smearing chocolate, honey, or whipped cream on each other and slowly licking it off. And for some, the taste of sex fluids is a total turn-on; for others a total turnoff. By now, it should be clear that if you allow your brain to get turned on, you will feel motivated to become sexually intimate with your partner. But if you are not turned on, there is no motivation for becoming sexual. If you decide to have sex when your brain is not turned on, you will not experience the total satisfaction of sexual pleasure. Don't get me wrong. It is quite possible to experience sexual activities without desire. You can feel exhausted from a hard day's work and all you want to do is climb into bed and sleep. You have zero desire. However, your partner begins to kiss your neck and bingo! Your sex centers spring into action and desire soars. What I am saying is that desire is essential if you want the greatest sexual experience possible.

Who Turns On Those Sex Centers?

If you are like most, you probably think that it is mostly up to your partner to stimulate your sex centers, right? Wrong! You are both responsible for keeping sex centers alive and well. I'm not saying that your partner doesn't give you a reason to turn on or off your sex centers, because that would be untrue. What I am saying, however, is even if your partner does give reason, you still have a choice whether or not you will keep your sex centers turned on or turn them off. You, and you alone, control your sex centers. Your partner, however, does contribute to your sex centers being on or off.

Let's take a closer look at how your thoughts and feelings come into play. Let's say that your desire is high because you had a sexy fantasy during the day about your partner. You, and you alone, have turned on your sex centers, right? After all, your partner wasn't even around when you entertained your fantasy. Now, he or she walks through the door and you are ready to jump their bones. However, something stupid is said, like, "You must have been busy today, you look a wreck." What happens? Yes, your sex centers just slammed shut.

Now, stop and think about this for a moment. I realize that your partner was the culprit, giving you a reason to turn off your sex centers. However, you are the one in charge of your brain and mind, not your partner. You have two choices: (1) you can powerfully discuss your hurt feelings with your partner and work it through. By making this choice you will keep your sex centers turned on; or, (2) don't tell your partner that this stupid comment hurt you, remain angry, and choose to keep those sex centers shut. I am sure you know that it is impossible to control your partner's behavior or actions. However, you can choose not to be a victim of anyone's inconsiderate behavior. Just like anything else in life, you are totally in charge of the outcome. The same holds true for sexual desire. Certainly, there will be various things in life that can cause a temporary loss of libido. However, you can ultimately make a choice as to how important having desire in your life is to your relationship.

Let's take a look at the two phases of desire.

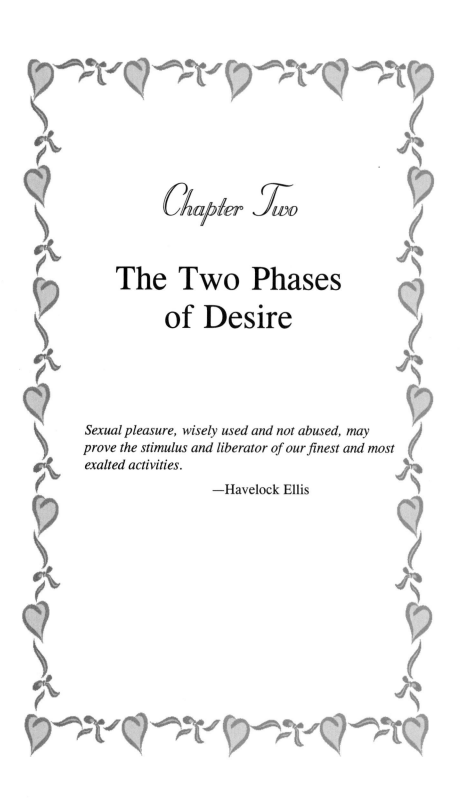

Chapter Two

The Two Phases
of Desire

Sexual pleasure, wisely used and not abused, may prove the stimulus and liberator of our finest and most exalted activities.

—Havelock Ellis

There are two distinct phases of desire. The initial phase, when two people first meet, is called euphoric lust. During this phase the sex centers seem to be on high alert. The couple doesn't have to work at keeping sexual desire high. Lust is present automatically. The second phase, when the couple has been together for a period of time, is enduring love. During this phase, the couple has to make some type of effort to keep those sex centers turned on.

Almost every couple I have seen in therapy has experienced these two phases. Yet, not being clear about making a distinction between the two can leave couples confused, hurt, and disappointed. Every relationship will go through the euphoric lust phase. However, not all relationships will enter the enduring love phase of love. In a moment, you will find out why.

Euphoric Lust

This is a phase of pure passion, in which two people who hardly know each other experience a heightened sexual desire and label this as falling in love. Euphoric lust is effortless; every waking moment is filled with thoughts of the other, and there is no question that the two will become sexually involved if there is the slightest opportunity.

The term lust, according to the *Oxford Dictionary,* is animal passion or desire. Most of us would have to admit that it is fun to be sexually animalistic at times, and lust is a great component to any relationship. If we are looking for a long-term relationship, however, we will need more than lust to sustain it.

You might say then that euphoric lust is an irrational, love-smitten phase that begs for an emotional connection with someone we hardly know. Does this sound irrational and crazy? You bet it is. To gain a deeper understanding of what euphoric lust is, let's use you as the example.

Do you remember when you initially fell in love with your partner? Can you remember the intensity of your feelings? Why did you fall in love with your partner? How much did you actually know about him or her that had you fall madly, passionately, and head over heels in love? Hardly anything, that's what! All you knew was that you were in love and wanted to become emotionally connected to this unknown person, and you desperately wanted this love returned.

Despite the intensity of these feelings, euphoric lust can also be exhausting. Why, you ask? Euphoric love plunges us into an intense physiological state. This state is manifested by blushing, perspiring, accelerated heart rate, butterflies in the stomach, and rapid breathing. There are some people who actually cannot eat, sleep, or concentrate. All they can think about is that person they hardly know. Remember the movie *Moonstruck*? In that movie, Nicholas Cage fell head over heels in lust with Cher. Even her slap didn't seem to make him snap out of it. Other people experience a heightened sense of well-being and vitality. Euphoric lust makes them feel happy, creative, and productive. Did you see the film *Shakespeare in Love*? The day that Shakespeare met the woman of his dreams, he wrote an entire play, *Romeo and Juliet,* which, by the way, is all about euphoric lust.

Euphoric lust can be a life-altering experience. I once treated a man who had been clinically depressed for over three years. He had been working in a law firm but hated being an attorney. Quite frankly, he hated his life. He met a woman on a skiing trip and fell madly in love, and she felt the same. Instantly, his depression lifted and he changed professions. Although their euphoric lust phase has ended, they are enjoying the lovely comfort of the second phase of enduring love.

What makes us choose that one particular person out of the hundreds of others we have met in our lives? It's a complex question that does not have a definitive answer. What we do know is that sexual attraction is totally subjective. What attracts one person may not attract another.

Euphoric lust does not last. However, its duration is different for everyone. For some, euphoric lust only lasts a couple of weeks, and for others it can last for a couple of years. One thing is certain, euphoric lust does end. Although many may find this phase exciting, the second phase is much more rewarding.

On the other hand, there are some people who enjoy this euphoric lust phase so much that they spend their entire lives going from one partner to the next in an effort to recapture that lustful experience. However, they never experience the type of love that being in a committed relationship brings. These individuals love the chase but hate the commitment. Many people live this way. There is nothing wrong with that, provided they remain single and they are honest with others about their particular lifestyle.

Why Do Most Individuals Enter This Euphoric Lust Phase?

The answer is twofold. Physically, it's nature's way of providing intense sexual desire that will lead to frequent sexual intercourse making procreation a possibility. Emotionally, it has us concentrate on all of our partner's positive traits and filters out the negative. Unfortunately, this often gets lost by the wayside when the couple gets comfortable with each other.

I'd like you to remember how life was with your partner during this initial phase. Those days were filled with passion and exciting love-making. There was intensity in every experience you shared. You overlooked each other's shortcomings, you thought of each other constantly, you laughed at each other's not always funny jokes, your heart would pound when you kissed, and you felt energized when together and lethargic when you were apart. You actually listened to each other and validated the other's point of view. You both shared your deepest and sometimes darkest secrets. You were inseparable. Most likely you both felt you were the most important, attractive, smart, and sexy person on the planet. You felt totally loved and valued.

Then something happened. You could feel a difference. Your heart didn't pound as hard when you were around one another, nor did you make love as often. You each stopped laughing at each other's not so funny jokes; and you each stopped actively listening to one another. You could almost feel euphoric lust coming to an end. It was as if you were being released from a spell. Some of you were relieved, and others were disappointed. Some of you actually thought that perhaps you were no longer in love. This is, of course, a misconception. Once you have experienced euphoric lust and it ends, you can recapture those feelings during the enduring love phase.

Enduring Love

Enduring love is the phase we can enter when euphoric lust ends. We are finally released from the craziness of this spell. Not all couples, however, make the decision to enter the enduring love phase. That's because the enduring love phase demands the final commitment to share in one another's lives.

As mentioned earlier, there are many people who hate the idea of being paired for life. They much prefer having several partners to keep euphoric lust alive. Others like the idea of sharing their life with a best friend and lover; for them, enduring love is quite appealing. Enduring love takes effort. Each partner must consciously invest energy in maintaining a healthy relationship, which includes sexual. But unlike euphoric lust, you will not feel as if you're at the mercy of those feelings. You will recapture all the positive and joyful aspects of euphoric lust, but without all of the craziness and lack of clear judgment.

Why Don't More Couples Decide to Enter the Enduring Love Phase?

There are four reasons that couples are hesitant about moving into the enduring love phase. First, most people hate relinquishing the fantasy that a perfect person exists. The couple is now faced with the stark reality of really getting to know one another without the use of blinders. Plus, they may not like what they discover. If euphoric lust is based on the qualities you think your lover has, then enduring love is based on the qualities you know your lover has—as well as what he or she doesn't have. When you commit to enduring love, you have to be willing to accept what you love about your partner as well as what might sometimes drive you crazy.

The second reason is because the enduring love phase is a lifetime commitment. Although most people say they want a lifelong relationship, many people get frightened when it comes to actually making that commitment.

The third reason is related to your level of willingness to put powerful energy into your relationship. To have a happy and enduring relationship requires continued hard work, and some just hate the idea of that much work, especially after experiencing the relative effortlessness of euphoric lust.

And the final reason is all about sex. In the enduring love phase, you cannot expect to be as overwhelmingly sexual as you both were during the euphoric lust phase. On the other hand, there is absolutely no reason why you cannot continue to feel wild desire for your partner. It just won't happen every second of every day. You certainly can enjoy lovemaking just as much, if not more than before. This phase allows you to explore the attributes and values that you feel are important for a lifelong partner.

What Are These Important Attributes and Values?

Most of us want our partners to possess attributes and values that we ourselves consider important and to have them closely matched to the ones we actually possess. These could include authenticity, honesty, trustworthiness, respectfulness, dependability, being demonstrative with affection and love, accepting of others who are different from us, being sexually responsive, self-disclosing, emotionally strong, humorous, intelligent, sincere, forgiving, spiritual, empathic, ethical, and powerful, just to name a few. What are the attributes and values you possess? What are the attributes and values you feel are important in your partner? For the most part, the person you are paired with is often a reflection of who you are. For some of us, this can be hard to see if we don't fully accept our own shortcomings as well as our strengths. I am sure that the majority of you have partners that are wonderful. You would not be reading this book if that were not true.

When we discover our partner's positive attributes and values, being sexual is one of the most beautiful ways of communicating just how much we love one another. Really, what can be more exquisite and giving? You are actually communicating on a deeper and more spiritual level, with your entire being, offering yourself totally to your partner, and accepting your partner's love is an act of total trust. When enduring love is at its best, neither of you cares much about fancy techniques or bothers asking yourself, "How am I doing? Am I doing this better than anyone else? Am I taking too long, or am I not lasting long enough?" You make love with every gesture and look, gently taking your partner's hand, enjoying a warm embrace and tender kissing, flirting during dinner, caressing one another in the bedroom, or taking long sensual bubble baths together. Enduring love is gloriously comfortable and secure.

Exercise: Getting to Know Each Other

This exercise is most likely one that you and your partner did not do prior to entering the enduring stage of love. Few couples did this unless they were involved in premarital counseling. Yet, getting to know the personal attributes and values of that person you are spending the rest of your life with is important, wouldn't you say? Okay, here we go. Face your partner and list what attributes and values you feel he or she possesses. Take turns telling each other why you consider these to be important to you. For example, if you feel dependability is an important attribute that your partner possesses, your statement could go something like this:

You: I love that you are so dependable. This is important to me because I'd never been able to depend on anyone but myself until I met you. It's a great feeling to know I can count on you for anything.

Your partner: You're dependable, too. It's so great to know that when you say you'll do something or be somewhere at a certain time, I'm certain you'll follow through.

Now it's your partner's turn to go next, and so on.

Your partner: I consider you honest. You've never lied to me about anything. I can totally trust that anything you do or say is true. I feel honesty is the most important value our relationship can have. I want to acknowledge you for your honesty.

You: Thanks. I also feel that honesty is important. Without it, I don't think I could remain in this relationship either. If you don't have honesty, I feel you can't have love or respect. I love your honesty.

Now that you get the picture, I'll let you continue on your own. This exercise should take about an hour. It is not only an exciting one, but it opens the door to great discoveries. If, however, your partner lists an attribute that you possess, but you do not feel he or she possesses it, but would like to see it developed, be authentic in your response without becoming angry. What is important is that you can let your partner know that it would be important to you if he or she works on developing this attribute.

The Meaning of Commitment

Commitment is promising to share your life with one another and to remain faithful. Although this can be a bit frightening, you have to admit it is also quite exciting. If your partner possesses attributes that you consider important and you both share a similar value system, why not? You are most likely partnered with your best friend. What can be nicer than sharing your life with your best friend?

A commitment does not necessarily mean a legal agreement either. There are thousands of couples who love one another and are committed without a legal document.

Commitment is also about putting your relationship first—not just in theory, but also in practice. This is where the work comes in, but that work can be fun once you get the hang of it. Some of you began a family, and your children became first priority. You began to deal with financial stresses, parental stresses, and pressures from your job. You were working wildly at the office putting in too many hours a week in an effort to save for your first home. Some of these everyday stresses began to take their toll on the relationship. You no longer felt like you were number one. You began to have small arguments that you did not have time to resolve. These unresolved arguments led to bigger ones. Finally, you felt so overwhelmed, disappointed, and angry, that you no longer even tried to resolve these issues. Needless to say, this negativity will certainly get in the way of sexual desire.

If you are married with children, what I'm going to say next will probably surprise you, but try to keep an open mind. Your relationship must take precedence over your children. This is not about being selfish; it is about keeping the best interests of your relationship and your children in mind. Consider this: if you put your children first rather than your relationship, your relationship will suffer. And if it suffers enough, you will wind up in divorce court. If you are divorced, the children will suffer this loss. Of course, I'm not suggesting that you ignore your kids. After all, you both made this decision to have children, and it is your responsibility to take good care of them. Besides, spending time with your children is deeply satisfying. All children need to be involved in family activities; it creates a sense of safety and security in childhood that leads to wonderful memories for them to treasure as adults. You both, however, need couple time without the kids at least once a week.

Okay, it's time for another exercise.

Exercise: A Walk Down Memory Lane

Face your partner and discuss exactly what commitment means to you. When did you make this decision to commit for a lifetime? Can you remember what you were thinking and feeling? For example, I made the commitment to spend the rest of my life with my partner when I watched him interact with my two very precious children. I knew if I could entrust my kids to have a relationship with him, he was definitely someone I wanted to share my life with. They also cared about him, and you know how perceptive children are. My partner told me he was also ready for a total commitment when he left us in Chicago to take a position at Johns Hopkins and could hardly stand the stress of a long-distance relationship. For me, total commitment meant having that marriage license. Hence, we got married. We continue to commit to each other on a monthly basis. For the past twenty-three years, we have had a monthly celebration on the date we met. This monthly recommitment is a nice way of validating our relationship.

Now it's your turn. Take that walk down memory lane. This exercise should take anywhere between thirty minutes and an hour.

Did you enjoy the walk? It's great to reactivate those old memories.

Let's move on. Now you know the true meaning of enduring love. But you should also be aware of the fact that you can both share important attributes, a similar value system, and be completely committed to your relationship and yet still fall prey to a sexual desire disorder. I will continue to mention that individual power and power reciprocity are the aphrodisiacs used to increase sexual desire. Exercising this power often can prevent a sexual desire disorder from occurring in the future.

The Dance between Your Mind and Desire

Now, let's take a look at how our brain and mind can either encourage or discourage sexual desire. An eloquent definition of this dance comes from a noted neuroscientist, Simon LeVay (1991), when he stated that the mind is just the brain doing its job.

I will give you an example of how the mind and desire work together. Let us say you have had a hard day at work or at home. You are tired and somewhat cranky from your difficult day, and the last thing on your mind is sex. Essentially, you are sending messages to the sex centers of your brain that you are not in the mood. These centers will remain shut down unless you tell them otherwise. Now, let's say that your partner has had a great day, is in the mood, and decides to create an ambiance conducive for intimacy. Fresh flowers, lighted candles, a drawn bubble bath, and a glorious dinner await you. You can perceive this circumstance in two very different ways; it's your choice.

The first way would be that you appreciate the romantic effort, but you inform your partner that you had a hellish day and you are too tired to make love. You would, however, enjoy the relaxation of a bubble bath, and you certainly appreciate the lovely dinner that is being presented. This keeps the sex centers on possible alert. After your luxurious bath, the two of you enjoy your dinner with an intimate, connected conversation and something wonderful begins to happen. The pressures of the day melt away and you are filled with energy and loving feelings. Those tired and sleepy sex centers are beginning to become activated. The two of you proceed into the bedroom, and your partner gently begins to remove your clothes and sweetly kisses your shoulders. The touch and kiss feel electric. Every inch of your body is turned on, and you return the touch and kisses. You begin to remove your partner's clothing, and the two of you continue to make love in a slow and sensuous manner that may eventually result in orgasm and possibly sexual intercourse. After lovemaking, the two of you embrace one another, until you finally sleep.

That is your brain and mind and that romantic circumstance at work. Even though you were initially exhausted from your day at work, you allowed your sex centers to be turned on by your own thoughts, feelings, and perceptions of this loving environment. If more partners made the effort to create such a romantic environment, there would be zillions of people making love more often. Keep in mind, however, that desire is the precipitation of romance, not vice versa.

The second way would be that you perceived this romantic scenario as a pressure to have sex, therefore keeping those centers shut down. In that situation you would drain the tub, blow out the candles, gobble down dinner, and get to bed early. Sure, you would get your much needed sleep, but you would also leave your partner feeling unappreciated, unloved, and most likely angry or disappointed.

Why do you think the outcomes of the same scenario were totally different? It is because your own thoughts are what turn the brain's sex centers on and off. But don't forget that your partner had a lot to do with either contributing to or interfering with sexual motivation.

A Tango between Circumstance and Desire

The notion that human beings can naturally have sex anytime with any-body is a myth. Some animals certainly can, but humans have evolved into thinking, feeling, and perceiving beings. That means our bodies and our minds must work together. The mind controls our thoughts, feel-ings, and fantasies, and interprets a particular circumstance prior to deciding whether or not to unleash desire or suppress it. The next illus-tration will play out exactly what I mean.

Imagine being in a room totally naked, and you are anxiously wait-ing for a particular someone to enter the room. In comes that person, who then begins to touch you all over your body. Are you going to allow your sex centers to be activated? No, not if that certain someone is your physician who is conducting an exam. See what I mean? If this same situation occurred with your partner in a romantic setting and your partner lovingly touched your body, your mind would allow those sex centers to turn on.

Here's another example. What if you and your partner were ready to make love but you heard your sick child crying in the other room? You would have the power to turn those sex centers off immediately, no matter how turned on you had been just a second ago. You, and only you, have the power to stop the brain's sex centers from reacting, even though the brain has experienced the activation of your sex centers. Or, let us say you are at a crowded beach, and you are turned on by your partner. It would be inappropriate to act on your desire—unless you are an exhibitionist and want to risk being arrested—so you will temporarily deactivate your sex centers at will, even if it takes a lot of will. But if you are at the beach at night, and there is no one around, you might decide to go skinny-dipping and make love in the water. As you can see, circumstance involves the right person, at the right time, in the right place, and the right occasion.

Does This Mean that I Have Total Power over My Sex Centers?

Yes, you do. Understanding that you have ultimate power to turn on or turn off those sex centers can be liberating. It can also, once and for all, dispel that old myth about how some people—and this is usually attributed to men—cannot control their lust when it comes to sexual temptation. I remember a couple who came into therapy because the husband had had an affair *only once,* and the wife was considering divorce. His excuse for this sexual fling was, "She pressed herself into me and grabbed my penis. I don't know a man on earth who could have resisted something like that. As soon as I came to my senses, I knew that I had made a huge mistake. My wife doesn't seem to understand that men can't resist such temptation."

Of course, I quickly brought to his attention that men and women do resist circumstances of temptation similar to the one described. I explained that our genitals do not make decisions; our mind, however, does. Men and women are continually subjected to sexual temptation. That does not mean that they give in to temptation and risk losing their partner. Unfortunately, this couple did get a divorce. She felt that if, by his own admission, he actually could not resist sexual temptation this *one time,* there would be hundreds of other temptations, to which he might also succumb. She simply could not live with someone that she could not trust.

Exercise: Measure Your Desire Level

The following questions are similar to the ones I ask my patients during sex therapy. Flip a coin to determine who will answer first. Face one another, read the questions, and then answer them out loud to one another. There are no right or wrong answers. Be honest and authentic. Remember, the more authentic and honest you are with one another, the more helpful this book will become in activating your sex centers.

The following questions require a yes or no answer. I realize that some of you may be somewhere in the middle. I do, however, want you to choose only a yes or no answer that fits most of the time, and then elaborate on your answer. To keep track of your answers, write them down, because after you read the entire book, I want you both to go back and do these exercises again sometime in the near future to see your progress. For heaven's sake, don't turn this into brain surgery. Have fun with this! I will give you an example of a typical answer to the first question.

- *Do you consider your partner romantic most of the time?*

You: Well, sometimes you are and sometimes you're
                   not. If I have to choose either yes or no, I'll have
                   to go with the no answer, because most of the
                   time you're not. Sorry honey, I don't want to hurt
                   your feelings, but I have to admit to you that I no
                   longer consider you romantic. You used to be. I
                   remember during our courtship days, when you
                   used to send me love notes all the time, but you
                   just don't do that anymore. I have to say that I
                   really miss that.

Your partner: I don't want to hurt your feelings either, but I'll
                   also have to go with no. You're right about our
                   courtship days. I remember one evening, when
                   you picked me up from work, and had a blanket,
                   a picnic basket loaded with cheese, oysters,
                   grapes, strawberries, chocolate, and other good-
                   ies hidden in the trunk of your car. You then
                   drove me to the lake without saying a word.
                   When we got to the lake, you whispered, "Sur-
                   prise." We got out of the car, spread out the blan-
                   ket, you lit several candles, and we proceeded to
                   dig into the picnic basket. It's a good thing we
                   didn't get caught skinny-dipping! Boy, was I ever
                   turned on. It was great. But we just don't take the
                   time to do those romantic things anymore. Maybe
                   it's time that we create more romance in our
                   lives.

Okay, it's your turn.

- *Does your partner show you affection most of the time?* In
  other words, does your partner gently kiss you, embrace you,
  hold your hand, rub your feet, stroke your hair, and so on,
  without these behaviors leading to sexual intercourse?

- *Is your partner attentive to you most of the time?* For example,
  if you have a headache, backache, a bad day at work or home,
  feeling blue, feeling edgy, and so on, is he or she sensitive and
  empathic regarding your needs?

- *Is your partner receptive/responsive to you when you are feeling like being sexual?* When you are in the mood does your partner readily accept your invitation for making love?

- *Do you consider you partner sexy?* Does your partner fit your idea of your sexual fantasy?

- *For the most part, can you turn yourself on sexually?* In other words, are you able to turn on your sex centers when the circumstances are conducive for lovemaking?

- *Do you personally feel that there is enough intimacy in your relationship?* Can you share your deepest secrets, concerns, dreams, wants, and needs with your partner?

- *Are you able to form sexual mental images (fantasies) prior or during lovemaking to jump-start your sex centers?* Can you picture you and your partner involved in an erotic, sexually charged scenario that you would not actually do in real life? For example, make love in a crowded elevator with hundreds of people watching, or ride on a horse naked through the streets of your town? You get the picture. Are you creative in your sexual fantasies?

- *For the most part, do you find being sexual with your partner a glorious experience?* Does your partner take enough time during foreplay to embrace, kiss, stroke your entire body, and stimulate your genitals? Are his or her sexual techniques perfect to the point that they need no improvement? Be gentle and sensitive in answering this question.

- *Are you and your partner sexually uninhibited enough to experiment with more creative and different sexual techniques and fantasies?* Do you both feel free and comfortable with one another to sexually experiment or are you too embarrassed or shy to try out new things?

- *Do you emphasize your partner's positive attributes?* If, for example, you see that your partner has put on some extra pounds, or lost some hair, or has a few more wrinkles, do you concentrate on these things or do you focus on things that you consider the most attractive attributes of your partner? In other words, do you emphasize the positive and ignore the negative?

- *Does your partner need to add an attribute or value that you consider important?* If so, tell your partner what you would like him or her to add.

- *Do you currently feel that your partner is attractive and fits your sexual fantasy?* If yes, explain to your partner all the physical features that you feel are so attractive. If no, gently explain this as well. For example, I used to smoke. My partner told me that this was a sexual turnoff because he feared for my life and he hated the way my breath smelled. Although it took me a long time to kick my addiction, I did brush my teeth before kissing him.

- *When your partner invites you to make love, do you usually agree?* I'm not talking about all the time, but most of the time.

- *Do you usually agree to make love because you really want to?* Do you make love because you don't want to hurt his or her feelings or do you really want to make love?

- *Do you feel that your sex drive is similar to your partner's?* Do you think your partner's sex drive is higher or lower than yours?

- *Do you feel sexual fantasies are healthy?* Do you feel that having fantasies is somehow improper?

- *Do you have sexual urges for your partner when you are away from one another?* Do you think about having sex with your partner, when he or she is at work?

- *When you are not in the mood, is it possible to be coaxed by a romantic ambiance?* Remember that example of the romantic dinner and bubble bath?

- *Do you masturbate?* Self-pleasuring is healthy and keeps those sex centers used to being activated. After all, your brain has to conjure up an erotic fantasy for erotic pleasure to take place.

- *Would you describe your relationship as an equal one?* In other words, do you make as many relationship decisions as your partner?

- *Do you know how to help your partner turn on his or her sex centers?* If not, ask for suggestions.

- *When you have experienced desire in the past, would you describe sexual activities as being exciting, rewarding, and fun?* For example, I had to explain to my partner that I hated talking during sexual activities. Maybe there's something that you would like to change as well.

- *Do you feel comfortable with your communication skills, including sexual?* In other words, do you connect on an intimate level when you talk to each other?

You now have tons of information about sexual desire. You've accomplished a lot of work. Please put the book down and take a well-deserved break. Now that you are both aware that you are and continue to be in the enduring love phase, the next step is to create an intimate boundary.

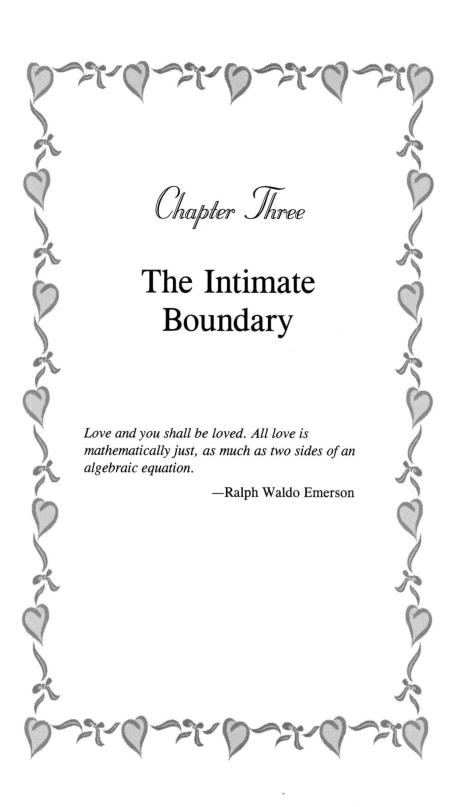

Chapter Three

The Intimate
Boundary

*Love and you shall be loved. All love is
mathematically just, as much as two sides of an
algebraic equation.*

—Ralph Waldo Emerson

The following is a typical scenario happening all over the world as we speak.

Partner A: Honey, why don't you come to bed?

Partner B: No thanks, I'm not sleepy, I think I'll read for a little while.

Partner A: I'm not inviting you to come to bed to sleep, I have other things we can do besides sleep.

Partner B: Honey, I'm not in the mood.

Partner A: You're never in the mood. You haven't been in the mood for weeks.

Partner B: I'm sorry, my days are exhausting and I just don't have the energy to make love.

Partner A: When will you have the energy to make love? Come on honey, it's been weeks.

Partner B: Please stop pressuring me. I'm simply not in the mood; can't you just accept that?

Partner A: No, I can't. There must be something that you can do to get yourself in the mood.

Partner B: It's not me, it's you. You don't connect to me anymore.

Partner A: I'm asking you to connect with me right now.

Partner B: You just don't get it. I don't feel that same connection that we used to have.

Sound familiar? Of course it does. We have all had this conversation at some point in our relationship. If you don't feel an intimate connection with your partner, the outcome will be a lack of sexual motivation. Quite simply, you can't get in the mood. It doesn't matter which one of you lacks this sexual desire. If it's you, your partner is equally responsible for this disconnection. If it's your partner, you are equally responsible. Both of you, however, are affected tremendously by the outcome and you both have to resolve this problem together.

Most couples scramble for possible solutions for their lack of desire. Couples arrive at the erroneous conclusions that perhaps they should incorporate novel techniques in their lovemaking. Or, perhaps romance is the key; perhaps they should try sex-enhancing products. Sure, it's great fun to tie each other up, or have dozens of candles glowing with flowers strewn everywhere, or each pop a Viagra. The truth is, however, that's not going to resolve anything. These props can come after you have the basics in place. What is the solution? Start over and learn the basics. The basics are the flame that heats up a relationship. That's what is exciting, exhilarating, and stimulating. You can experience your relationship as if it's brand-new.

It's going to be a fun process to rediscover your partner in a new light, and the results will be amazing. Are you ready? Buckle up, this will be a fast and thrilling ride! You are about to rediscover each other by learning the first basic component essential to your relationship.

Your Couple Boundary

While attending social events, I try to guess which two people are involved in an intimate boundary. What can I say, it's an occupational hazard. What do I look for? I look for two people who are holding hands, standing close together, looking intently into each other's eyes, or smiling at each other. There appears to be some type of aura around them that defines them as a couple. You can tell that they enjoy being in each other's company.

Then, there are other couples who appear to be disconnected. You know the type, one partner is on one side of the room, and the other is on the opposite side. Unless you had prior knowledge that they are involved, you would hardly guess that they were a couple. You can bet there is something missing in their relationship. What they lack is an intimate boundary.

Having a boundary around your relationship is vitally important, because it enhances intimate connection. If you cannot connect in the kitchen, you cannot connect in the bedroom. If I saw you and your partner in public, would I be able to tell that you were a couple? Hopefully, I would. If, however, I could not distinguish you as a couple, let's remedy this right now.

What Is a Couple Boundary?

A couple boundary is an invisible circle that surrounds the two of you. You automatically had this boundary in the beginning of your relationship, but you were, most likely, unaware of its existence. Remember those days? You were like magnets drawn to each other. The two of you were inseparable. Then, all of a sudden, it was no longer there. You could feel it. Something changed. There was a disconnection, but words could not explain what happened or why this happened. Confusion set in. You always assumed that as the relationship moved on in years, the intimacy would deepen. The opposite seems to be true. It seems you were more connected when you barely knew each other. How could that be?

The answer is that in the past, you both wanted a boundary placed around you. You loved the idea of being coupled, and you wanted others to acknowledge you as a couple. You either consciously or unconsciously made a decision to place this boundary around yourselves, but as time went on you allowed it to weaken. It's time to create a new and more powerful one.

How Do We Create a Couple Boundary?

A boundary is extraordinarily easy to create. All you have to do is draw an invisible circle around the two of you and act as a unit. The hard part is keeping this boundary intact. You have to protect it from breaking down.

Why Do We Need This Boundary?

There are four major reasons:

1. A boundary acts like a barrier protecting your relationship from outside intrusion.

2. A boundary forces you to develop rules that govern your relationship.

3. A boundary makes you cognizant of the fact that you function as a unit.

4. A boundary encourages a powerful, connected conversation that increases sexual desire.

What Can Cause a Breakdown of Our Boundary?

There are two types of forces at play that can unwittingly lead to the breakdown of your boundary, and ultimately to the breakdown of your sexual lives. These are external and internal forces. An external force is when you allow anything or anybody to interfere in your relationship. An internal force is when you and your partner cannot or will not agree on certain rules that govern your relationship.

It goes without saying, if your boundary is currently missing, there is nothing to either build on or protect. Let's take care of that right now and rebuild a new and more powerful boundary.

The Creation of Your Protected Barrier

Typically, two individuals have to be free and clear of their families of origin before they create their own couple boundary. That's not to say that you don't love your parents or you don't have an emotional connection to them, because that would be untrue. What I am stating is that you each have to cut the cord. You cannot allow your parents to interfere with or intrude on your personal relationship. You are probably thinking, "Come on, I haven't let my parents tell me what to do since I was sixteen years old." Well, I'm not so sure about that. Most couples have privately complained of external pressures on their relationship from their in-laws or an overbearing parent. It might surprise you how most couples I see do have boundary issues involving their families of origin. If you truly don't have these issues, that's great. You have successfully completed the initial task of creating your couple boundary. If you have experienced this external force at play and it interferes with your own relationship, read on.

Typical examples of external parental intrusion include three facets: advice giving, demands on time, and family tradition.

1. **Advice Giving.** I'm amazed at the millions of times I've heard couples start sentences off with, "His mom thinks we should buy a bigger house." Or, "My dad said that we should be investing in stocks." Or, "Our parents think it's time for us to start having children." Or, "Our parents hate the name we chose for our

baby, so we have to come up with another name." Or, "My dad wants me to return to law, instead of owning a coffee shop." Or, perhaps this advice giving runs even deeper: "I don't think you should be drinking wine every night; your dad and I only drank wine on Saturdays." Or, "You spend your money on the most frivolous things; you'll never have enough for retirement." Or, "Don't let Timmy suck on that pacifier, it will ruin his teeth." These statements go on ad nauseam.

You and your partner alone have the right to make any and all decisions relating to your relationship. That's why it is vitally important to develop a boundary. With your boundary in place, you have the right to respond to these statements as follows, "We don't want a bigger house." Or, "We would rather invest in real estate." Or, "We don't want children." Or, "We'll choose our child's name." Or, "Maybe you liked law but I like my coffee shop."

If, however, you ask for parental advice, that's a different story. But if you do not make a request for their advice and these well-intentioned individuals intrude, respectfully and lovingly keep them out of your boundary.

2. **Time Demands.** I am certain that most of you have parents and siblings who love you and want to spend time with you. That's great, but you have to set limits. It is essential that you and your partner spend quality time together. An example of this is Don and Nora. Don complained that Nora spent almost every Saturday morning with her sister, discussing a business venture. When he brought his complaint to Nora, she said, "We're with each other all week! Can't you be away from me for a couple of hours a week?" Don's point was that he felt Nora's sister was intruding on the their weekend time. He was right. Nora's sister was an external force who was unwittingly impinging on their boundary. It was up to Nora to figure out an alternate plan to see her sister for these business discussions. Perhaps an alternative could be that they meet over lunch during the workweek, rather than the weekend.

Very often, family members can make demands on your time at the expense of your relationship. Although they love you, these time demands can lead to problems. Here is another illustration of how time demands can inadvertently interfere with your sex centers. Tom and Tara have been living together for six months. Prior to their moving in together, they had an active sex life. For the past month, however, Tara has lost all sexual desire for Tom. It seemed that Tom's mother phoned him every evening to discuss the "events of the day." Tara felt Tom was confiding in his mother, rather than in her, and was feeling left out. It was fortunate, however, that Tara was able to openly address these unhappy feelings with Tom. Tom acted on Tara's feelings and explained to his mom that these nightly conversations were taking time away from him and Tara. He offered an alternative that both he and Tara could live with. He would briefly converse with his mom once a week, during his working hours. Due to this relatively simple change, Tom and Tara had the time needed for engaging in connected conversations, and that led to the restoration of Tara's sexual desire.

Many loving parents and siblings are unwittingly intrusive. It's up to you to gently inform them that your first priority is your relationship. Finding creative compromises is empowering to your relationship and reminds your partner of just how important they are to you.

3. **Traditions.** For most couples, holidays can be a nightmare. Most couples I know usually have two holiday dinners. You know who you are; you are both caring, loving people who are afraid of hurting your parents' feelings by not sharing the holidays with them. I think it is great to be that generous, as long as it does not intrude on your relationship. If, however, one of you would rather stay home for the holidays, you have a right to do just that. Gently and lovingly explain to them that you would like to start your own tradition by having your holiday dinner by yourselves or with friends. Or, perhaps there can be a compromise that you can all live with.

One of the most volatile discussions I had ever witnessed involved this couple who were arguing about when to open Christmas presents. He always opened his gifts Christmas morning, and she opened hers on Christmas Eve. It was humorous to watch them get so passionate about a tradition. They finally settled it by a compromise. One year they would open gifts in the morning, and the next year in the evening.

Whatever traditions you and your partner would like to implement, you have a right to do so free and clear of external intrusion. It's up to you and your partner to determine what works for your unique relationship.

Exercise: Lovingly but Firmly Keep Them Out

Sit facing one another and discuss incidents where parents or other family members unwittingly became intrusive. Come up with at least five examples. Come on, you are not betraying any love for your family members. What you are doing, however, is accomplishing the first task needed to develop your intimate boundary, and that is to keep them out.

Rules to Love By

Another reason for developing a boundary is that it helps define the rules that govern your own unique relationship. It forces you and your partner to make the compromises necessary to have your relationship run smoothly. For example, when you were single, you had certain rules that governed your own behavior. The most obvious is the freedom to have sex with as many partners as you choose. After you entered your current relationship, however, that rule most likely changed to one of monogamy and fidelity. Breaking this rule will no doubt cause problems in your relationship.

But what about the less conspicuous rules that governed you when you were single? Maybe you had dinner with your parents every Sunday. Or, you went out with friends every Saturday. Or, you joined your colleagues for a drink every night after work. These rules could possibly interfere with the functioning of your relationship. Take, for example, the fact that you or your partner would like to continue to have dinner with your folks every Sunday. Neither of you is free, however, to make this decision individually. This would require a conversation with your partner to see if it's okay with him or her. Perhaps you'll create a rule that you'll spend most of your Sundays dining alone as a couple.

As you can see, your couple boundary is important, because it forces you both to compromise and create new rules that are mutually acceptable. Yet, most couples have never actually sat down to have a conversation regarding new rules that govern their relationship. Flexibility and common sense are key when designing rules.

There are zillions of possible rules that can govern a relationship. Some rules will be permanently fixed, and others will change as your relationship changes. For example, let's say that one of your rules is that you equally share in the cooking, laundry, and household chores. Then, at some point in time, one of you gets laid off from your job. If one of you remains home all day, wouldn't it make sense to revise this rule? Maybe, maybe not. It is up to both of you to decide. Most importantly, if one of you does not like a rule, then it cannot be a success. The cardinal rule of a boundary is compromise.

Exercise: Let's Design Rules

Sit facing each other. Design at least five rules that will be part of your relationship. Make sure that these rules are important enough to warrant implementation. When having this conversation, keep in mind that the vitality of your relationship depends on the rules you create as a couple. Your relationship must always take top priority.

Together but Separate

Acting as a unit but simultaneously maintaining one's individuality seems confusing to most people. On the one hand, there are those individuals who are terrified of losing their identity within a relationship. Although they have their own boundary in place, they refuse to place one around their relationship. They guard their identity with all their might. These are the couples mentioned earlier who you would never guess are involved in a relationship. These couples are referred to as being disengaged.

On the other hand, there are those individuals who have not developed their own identity and lack an individual boundary to begin with. As a couple, they seem to meld together and appear to be joined at the hip. If I were to ask one of them, "How are you feeling today?" the other would answer and vice versa. These couples are enmeshed.

Let's briefly take a look at disengaged and enmeshed couples.

The Disengaged Couple

These couples, albeit rare, may sleep in separate bedrooms, take separate vacations, have separate friends, and seem to place their own individual needs over that of the relationship. I am sure you have noticed this type walking down the street. One of them is two feet ahead of the other. They are totally disconnected. There is a certain roommate quality to their relationship. They do, however, engage in sexual activities, but desire is missing. Hence, sex is typically ho-hum.

Are these couples doomed to leading separate lives without the benefit of a connection? No, of course not. Once they each realize that they will not have to relinquish their own sense of identity, they can relax and begin the movement necessary towards creating an intimate boundary.

The Enmeshed Couple

For the enmeshed couple, one or both individuals have no sense of identity and try to become what they think the other person wants them to be. They become overly involved in each other's lives. Instead of sharing a life with each other, they live their lives for each other. There is a certain brother-sister quality to their relationship. Obviously, if they *become one* identity, there isn't any type of tension, including sexual. When they engage in sexual activities, they are overly concerned with the other's pleasure. Well, if this happens, you shut off your own sex centers pretty quickly. Sex is pretty dull.

Are these couples doomed to a sibling relationship? No, not if they are willing to develop their own individual sense of self. Once this is accomplished, they can begin to put some separation between them and move towards creating a healthy boundary.

The Healthy Couple

The healthy couple has a little of both extremes. Each individual maintains their own identity and, at the same time, each is invested in the other's welfare. There can, however, be this unconscious wish for sameness, but not to the extreme of enmeshed couples.

I'll give you an example. Just for a minute, imagine yourself as a red ball of clay and your partner as a blue ball of clay. Initially, when you first met, you fell in love with his "blueness" and your partner loved your "redness." You each fell in love with the other's unique color. It would be pretty boring if you were both the same, wouldn't it? Over time, the most peculiar thing happens. All of a sudden, you want your partner to be a little more "red" like you, and your partner wants you to be a little more "blue" like him! The very color that you each once found so unique, you want to change. So, what happens when a red ball of clay and a blue ball of clay get mixed together? Pretty soon you don't know where your red starts or your partner's blue ends. You both can turn into a boring gray ball of clay.

There can also be the pretense for separateness that healthy couples manifest, but not to the extreme of disengaged couples. For example, for some crazy reason that I do not quite understand, men and women have this social ritual or celebration marking the end of their freedom, prior to getting married. I'm not quite sure if it's an excuse to see a male or female jump out of a cake buck naked, or what. The unconscious message, however, is that developing a couple boundary means the end of freedom and the beginning of imprisonment. Good grief, what kind of message is that! Last week, we attended a party where one of the guests had recently married. I approached him to congratulate him. He responded, "Yep, the old ball and chain is sitting over there." I said, "Oh, I'm so sorry for you. Do you view your partner as your jail warden?" His face turned beet red, and he said, "Of course not, I was just kidding around." I considered that to be an extremely negative mental image he projected. If he continued to think in those terms, he would eventually believe that a relationship means imprisonment, rather than the exhilarating feeling of sharing a life together. Be very, very careful of the words you choose. Language is powerful. If you give yourself a negative thought, eventually a similar feeling will follow. Unfortunately, this young man who was "just kidding around" was well on his way to disengagement if he didn't rid himself of this negative cognition.

Now that you understand the importance of developing an intimate boundary, I'd like to ask you this question: Would I be able to identify you and your partner as a couple at a social gathering? I bet I would.

Congratulations! You and your partner have created an intimate boundary that surrounds the two of you and defines you as a couple. Cherish it always.

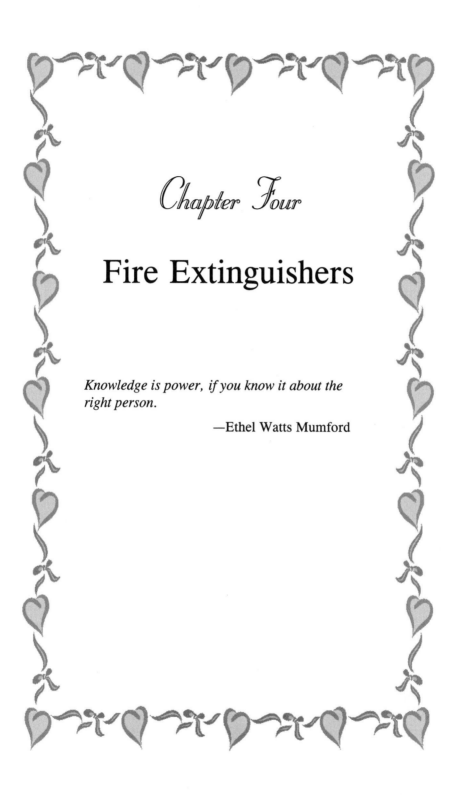

Chapter Four

Fire Extinguishers

*Knowledge is power, if you know it about the
right person.*

—Ethel Watts Mumford

A fire extinguisher is an interrelationship obstacle that has the potential of turning off your sex centers. As you are aware, if your sex centers are turned off, the result will be a diminished libido. In this chapter, you will be able to identify precisely when your relationship began to lose its sexual excitement. Once we examine all the factors that led to your drop in libido and figure out exactly how your situation brought about this dilemma, then, and only then, can we take the steps to resolve them. It would not make sense to rush you into fixing a problem unless you have a clear understanding of what needs fixing to begin with.

I cannot stress this enough; a lack of sexual desire is *not* simply an individual problem, it's a relationship one. There was something that happened or some obstacle that caused passion to wane. It is impossible to address each and every obstacle, because there are thousands. We can, however, take a look at the most common ones. By identifying the most prevalent ones and illustrating how they can be dealt with, you and your partner will be able to remove any obstacle that is hurting your own relationship. Keep in mind that the removal of any obstacle is only the first step in clearing the way towards ameliorating hypoactive sexual desire disorder; it's not the long-term cure.

Interrelationship obstacles do not, in and of themselves, necessarily lead to a lowered or diminished libido. At their core, however, are the negative thoughts and feelings of powerlessness that can pour ice-cold water on passion. If the obstacle is addressed immediately, free of the long-term negativity, the sex centers can be turned on.

Let's take a look at the most common of the interrelationship obstacles.

Inequality within a Relationship

Surely, most of us no longer buy into that tired old notion that men are supposed to "bring home the bacon" and women are supposed to keep the house clean and raise the kids. Come on now, we are much more evolved than that.

Don't get me wrong; I'm not being condescending about a traditional relationship where a woman works at home and is primary caretaker of the children, while the man is the financial provider. This situation is great as long as this decision was mutually agreed upon.

Nor am I putting down a less common relationship, where these roles are reversed. If this is a decision that you both have agreed to, there is absolutely nothing wrong with this arrangement. There are, however, many couples who have not had an explicit agreement. Instead, there was an implicit understanding that "that's the way things are supposed to be."

An example of this is Jack and Jill. They have been married for seven years and have a two-year-old named Sara. Jill lost total sexual desire for Jack one year ago. If she continues to refuse his sexual advances, he plans to seek a divorce. Jack loves Jill deeply but cannot accept a sexless marriage. Jill loves Jack but feels zero desire and doesn't know what to do to increase it. Let's take a look at how their relationship unraveled due to relationship inequality.

When they first met, Jill was a highly successful stockbroker, and Jack was an attorney with a successful law firm. For the first four years of marriage, they had an extremely active sex life. They made love every night, and sometimes twice a day during their weekends. They were elated when Jill became pregnant. Jill wanted to stay home and care for Sara, which they both agreed was a great idea. Jill's role, as primary caretaker, was extremely rewarding. After the end of two years, however, Jill wanted to return to work part-time. She told Jack that she was considering a return to work. He became enraged. He told her, "It's out of the question; we don't need the extra money, and our daughter needs a full-time mother! I refuse to have Sara raised by a stranger. Look at what's happening to children today. They are out of control, and most are on drugs. That's because mothers are not staying at home and taking care of them. You will not go back to work. I absolutely forbid it."

Jill was stunned by Jack's reaction. She told Jack, "Don't be ridiculous. Sara has two parents who love her deeply. That will not change. It's not the quantity but the quality of time spent connecting with children that's important. We can both interview candidates together and choose the best woman we feel will offer excellent care. I need to return to work because I need the intellectual stimulation of being around adults."

Jack insisted that it was important for the parent to provide care, not some stranger. Jill said, "If you think it's so important for a parent to be around a child all day long, why don't you quit your job and stay home with Sara, and I'll take care of the family finances." Jack was livid. "Men go to work. Women stay home and take care of kids. That's the way it's always been, and that's the way I want it! If it was good enough for our parents, it should be good enough for us."

Although Jill was equally furious, she felt powerless to do anything about the situation. She stayed home, but her resentment toward Jack manifested itself by a drop in her libido. Jack made several attempts to connect emotionally with Jill, phoning her during the day to tell her how much he loved her, hiring a housekeeper to clean the house, planning romantic weekends, taking her out for elaborate dinners, and surprising her with flowers and gifts. Although she appreciated this attention, his attempts were fruitless. Jill's sexual desire remained unmoved. She explained that she could hardly bring herself to kiss him when he returned from work each evening. Jack felt powerless, rejected, and unloved. He had no idea why Jill no longer felt like making love, and Jill couldn't understand why she no longer felt any sexual desire. That's when they entered couple therapy.

I wish I could offer you a happy ending; however, I can't. Although they finally understood that the obstacle interfering with sexual desire was inequality within their relationship, they could not remove it. Jack admitted that he was controlling the relationship but refused to change it. Jill understood that her anger and resentment caused her to develop a full-fledged hypoactive sexual desire disorder. He held on to his position that women should remain at home and men should be responsible for the finances. Jill refused to accept Jack's position and requested a divorce. Jack finally agreed. They currently have joint custody of Sara.

The irony of this situation is that both Jack and Jill are working full-time and were forced to hire outside care for Sara anyway. It's a shame that such a loving couple had to end their marriage because of inequality.

This next obstacle appears to be harmless, but it can lead to a desire disorder.

Flirtatious Behavior

Most of us can easily identify this obstacle. If your partner is flirtatious, you can probably pinpoint the exact second flirting began. There is nothing inherently wrong with flirting. Actually, it's fun and harmless if you are *not* involved in a committed relationship. However, within a loving relationship, it will often have negative consequences.

Although flirting usually does not end a relationship, it can lead to resentment, anger, distrust, and contempt. These negative feelings and thoughts are certainly desire busters. Think about the last time that your partner flirted with another person, or imagine yourself in that situation. Now, ask yourself how this made you feel. Did you feel embarrassed that your flirtatious partner needed the attention of another person? Did you feel angry? Did you feel insecure? Did you feel that others viewed you with sympathy and with secret relief that it wasn't their partner doing the flirting? Did you feel ridiculous that you felt powerless to do anything about this flirting? Did you doubt your own internal perceptions and feel that you were overreacting? Did you try to ignore what was going on? If you answered yes to any or all of these questions, you know that these negative thoughts and feelings lead to anger, contempt, distrust, and resentment. And, of course, this negativity will shut down the sex centers.

For those who feel that flirting is harmless fun, let me assure you that it's not. Flirting has only one motive: to solicit and receive sexual attention. Flirting does not, however, have to lead to physical sexual activity. But please, don't try to fool yourself. The thought of sexual activity is always present during flirtatious behavior.

I have heard every excuse in the book for *harmless* flirting. Here are examples of a few of my all-time favorites: My partner does not pay enough attention to me, so I need the attention of others. I love it when my partner feels jealous; it proves he or she loves me. It shows my partner that I'm attractive to the opposite sex. It means nothing; I just like doing it. It's fun and makes me feel that I'm still desirable. Who me? I don't flirt. Why are you so insecure? I'm just being friendly.

If you are flirtatious, remember that you are hurting your partner, even if you consider your flirting to be harmless. If your partner accuses you of being a flirt but you feel you are not flirtatious, what should you do? Ask yourself the following question: Why would my partner accuse me of flirting? The answer is, your partner is hurt by the attention that you are paying to others. Then ask yourself, Why on earth do I need this attention? Individuals who flirt might as well wear a neon sign around their neck that reads, "I am insecure; please pay attention to me." If your partner has accused you of flirting, please take responsibility for this inappropriate behavior and stop it.

If, however, you continue to flirt, the outcome is mostly the same. Your partner will feel resentment, anger, and contempt, even if he or she tells you, "It really doesn't bother me; I'm secure in who I am." Trust me, that statement is a cover-up for not wanting to appear jealous.

For those of you who cannot distinguish between being friendly and being flirtatious, I will list a few behaviors to help you to identify how a flirtatious individual behaves. Once distinguished, you'll have no more excuses. Keep in mind that flirting involves a willing and equally flirtatious recipient. Otherwise, it can be considered sexual harassment.

Identifying Flirtatious Behavior

- *When you pull out your seductive voice.* You know what I mean. It's a different voice that you would not normally use when speaking to your accountant about a tax audit.

- *When you move into another's personal space.* Most of us prefer around two feet that separates us from another. When you move closer, it's an unconscious wish for intimacy.

- *Directly or indirectly mentioning any type of sexual topic during a conversation.* I once heard a female describe to a male colleague an uncomfortable gynecological exam. She told him that while her legs were in the stirrups, she felt the physician was sexually exploiting her. Give me a break! Whether the physician was or was not a creep is not in question. When another person speaks, we automatically form mental pictures during the conversation. This male colleague must have formed some whoppers. She was definitely flirting, and he engaged in it by not ending this conversation. He was definitely enjoying his images.

- *Touching another gently.* I've watched this behavior occur between people who scarcely know each other. They are engaged in conversation, and one touches the other on the arm, hand, hair, or shoulder. Or, you're seated at a table, and someone's leg touches yours. I'm not talking about two friends who touch each other. I'm talking about touching when both individuals are aware it's a sexual touch. You get the picture.

- *Complimenting someone on how he or she looks.* "Oh, you look so handsome in that tie." Of course the tie has tiny smiley faces all over it. Or, "Wow, you look spectacular in that dress." Of course the dress is the one you wore to your grandmother's funeral. Again, I'm not talking about an honest compliment.

- *Penetrating or wandering eye contact.* You know that look. A flirt is so painfully obvious. He or she will continue to watch your mouth or other body parts. Usually a flirt will know exactly with whom they can do this.

Now, let's take a look at a new type of sexual activity that is sweeping the nation. Internet sex. What starts out as innocent fun in the chat room can end a relationship.

Computer Sex

Ah, the joys of modern technology. Computers have revolutionized and enhanced our lives beyond belief. Technology, however, can present certain problems that concern many therapists today. The major concern is that computers are replacing face-to-face relationship discussions. I am personally witnessing more and more couples destroy their relationships because of the problems created by entering chat rooms.

Here is an example of how harmless fun can ruin relationships. Dan and Linda have been involved in a relationship for over eight years. Dan stated that four months ago Linda was out of town and, out of boredom, he entered a chat room. He became involved in a conversation with a woman regarding politics. He found this conversation exciting and insightful.

Linda worked nights as a physician. This situation afforded Dan the opportunity to converse with his new on-line friend. Dan started to look forward to having these conversations. These chats, however, began to slowly change from data sharing (informational) to more intimate (connected) ones. He felt safe with this flirtation because of the anonymity involved. After a few weeks, they revealed their true identities as well as phone numbers. This flirtation gradually turned into graphic sexual conversations. Then it happened. They replaced computer sex with phone sex. Their relationship took on a new form of intimacy: hearing one another's voices.

After months of what Dan considered harmless fun, his computer pal took it to a new level. She professed her love (euphoric lust) for him and wanted to get married! Dan was stunned, and quickly stated that he was involved in a committed relationship with Linda. The woman became enraged. She accused Dan of leading her on. She phoned Dan constantly, begging him to end his relationship with Linda. When Dan refused, she phoned Linda and revealed her identity. Linda was shocked, hurt, and angered by the fact that Dan could betray her in this manner. Dan denied any wrongdoing, because he didn't actually engage in physical sex. Dan's denial further enraged Linda. Although he promised never to enter a chat room again, Linda's resentment, anger, and disappointment did not lift, which resulted in hypoactive sexual desire disorder. Fortunately, they learned how to tap into power and their relationship was happily restored.

I've also seen computer sex go to a higher level yet. After following the process explained, some decide to physically meet and have sex. This brings us to the next obstacle that, unfortunately, is quite common.

Infidelity

Contrary to popular belief, both men and women are just about equal in committing infidelities. Although men think it's mostly a male behavior, it's not.

Studies show that most men commit an infidelity because lust and novel sex were missing from their relationship. In contrast, most women seek out an affair because intimacy was lacking in their relationship.

When there is betrayal within the relationship, it's an understatement to say that this will lead to a turnoff of sex centers. When you are lied to and deceived, it would be ridiculous to think you would want to make love with someone who could hurt you so badly. You are probably wondering if a relationship can be restored if the couple boundary has been violated. The answer is yes; however, it takes much hard work to restore trust.

A Libido Discrepancy

Most couples have a libido discrepancy. A libido discrepancy means that one partner wants to have sex more frequently than the other. A classic example of a libido discrepancy is a scene from one of Woody Allen's movies, *Annie Hall*. Woody's therapist asks how often he and his partner are having sex. He says, "Hardly ever; two times a week." In the next scene, his partner, played by Diane Keaton, is asked the same question by her therapist, and she answers, "All the time; two times a week." This perception is common; it happens frequently. What's important is that these differences in perception are discussed with one another.

The primary danger of a libido discrepancy is that the partner requesting sex may feel rejected, misunderstood, confused, angry, and unloved. The requested partner can feel sexually inept or feel like a sex object. When you have these feelings and they are not discussed, sexual desire in either or both partners can take a nosedive.

What is normal sexual frequency? It's what you and your partner say it is. You both, however, will have to compromise. If, for example, you are happy with once a month but your partner wants sex daily, what then? Engage in a powerful discussion to determine what you can each live with. You would certainly have to pick up your pace, and your partner would have to lower the pace considerably. If you or your partner has a high sex drive, my suggestion is to masturbate more frequently. It's not as much fun as sex with your partner, but it can be just as satisfying.

Not Being Able to Engage in Sexual Fantasy

This obstacle is extremely important. A sexual fantasy is a mental process that represents our most passionate sexual desires and wishes. Fantasies are healthy and fun. A fantasy can be used to jump-start your sex centers. Without these mental representations, it's difficult to turn on sex centers.

Although everyone has the ability to have fantasies, most women experience guilt, because they somehow feel that their fantasies are either inappropriate or they feel like they are cheating if they involve a male other than their husband. I want to reassure you that it's not cheating; it's a fantasy, that's all. Unlike phone and computer sex, which are not fantasies but sexual behaviors, few women have acted on their fantasies. After all, the likelihood of a sexy movie star walking through your door anytime soon is slim. And even if he did, you'd have the choice of saying, "No thanks, I'm involved in a committed relationship."

Most studies, however, show that the primary star of our fantasies is our partner. It can be so much fun if you act out a fantasy with your partner. I had a male patient who was afraid of telling his wife that he fantasized that she was a streetwalker when he made love to her. This totally turned him on. However, he was ashamed of this fantasy and had tried for years to make it go away. I asked him, did he truly, in real life, consider his wife a whore? He laughed and said, "Of course not."

I then asked him if he thought his wife would think he thought of her as a streetwalker if he shared his fantasy with her. He replied, "Of course not." I suggested that he share this fantasy with her. He took my suggestion and told her of his fantasy. She laughed and said, "Hey, would you like me to dress up like one tonight?" He gladly accepted her invitation. She told me that she had a lot of fun getting dressed for the part and got totally turned on. He said she looked great, but he certainly would not want her to leave the house looking like that. They not only had fun with his fantasy, but also experienced fireworks in bed that evening. Fantasies are fun with the person you love, trust, and respect. Be creative; however, *never* engage in anything that makes you feel uncomfortable.

A word of caution: Use your common sense when it comes to sharing a fantasy. I once told a couple to share their favorite fantasies. The woman told her partner that her favorite fantasy was making love to his brother. Needless to say, I almost fainted. I had to develop a pretty creative intervention to get her out of that! Share only the fantasies that include your partner. Our next obstacle includes everyone.

Everyday Stress

If you are alive, you will experience stress. Common stressors can include financial difficulties, being a parent, taking care of an elderly parent, being fired from a job, looking for a job, the loss of a loved one, going through invasive infertility treatment, a divorce, or a move. The list goes on and on. Couples can experience sheer exhaustion as a result of these stressors. This fatigue can temporarily turn off those sex centers. After all, if all you can think about is getting some well-deserved rest, you will not feel like making love. Why not take a short vacation? Take a breather from the everyday routine. You deserve it.

If, however, these stressors become chronic, you may be at risk for experiencing a sexual desire disorder. This requires more drastic measures. This means that you must put your own needs in front of everyone else's. Every day you must take at least one hour for meditation or relaxation. Get a massage, go to a movie, take a walk, sink into a hot bubble bath, work out physically, lie down and clear your mind of all the daily minutiae, watch TV, read a book, practice relaxation techniques (tighten and relax you muscles), or eat an apple. When your mind and body feel relaxed, your sex centers are more amenable to receiving and returning love. Remember, it's impossible to experience stress and calmness at the same time.

Negative Body Image

As you already know, you and you alone have the power to turn on your sex centers. It's essential to desire to view yourself as attractive. It's not being conceited or narcissistic, it's just part of having healthy self-esteem. If you don't like the way you look, you will automatically trigger negative thoughts about yourself. Negative cognitions will always suppress sexual desire. Therefore, do whatever it takes to begin to appreciate your body. Love it and take good care of it. I will address negative body image in detail later in the book.

Boring Sexual Techniques

Let's face it, if your sexual techniques are starting to get boring, or they are not that creative to begin with, sexual desire can suffer. After all, sex needs to be fun and exciting for you to desire it. I'm not suggesting that you and your partner have to experiment with novel techniques if you are both satisfied with your current ones. Don't fix what isn't broken. If, however, you or your partner would like to experiment with new techniques, you will have to discuss this with one another. Most couples are too embarrassed to discuss sex with one another. Once you remove the shame and embarrassment regarding sexual discussions, you and your partner can be free to be more sexually creative. Desire is activated when you recall an exciting past sexual experience involving each other. This leaves you wanting more.

Unpleasant Sexual Techniques

If you and your husband, for example, decide to experiment with a novel sexual technique, such as anal sex, and you find this experience unpleasant, recalling this will shut down your sex centers. Never engage in a sexual technique that you consider unpleasant. Instead, explain to your partner that you disliked this experience and you never want to participate in this type of sexual activity again. If you don't have this conversation, you will be fearful that he'll attempt to repeat it in the future. This fear can keep your sex centers turned off.

Now, I want you to begin to think about the possible factors within your relationship that may be causing your sex centers to shut down. You may be surprised to learn that the obstacles that you feel exist might be different from those your partner mentions.

Exercise: Pinpoint Your Obstacles

Are you ready to pinpoint those obstacles interfering with sexual desire? Face one another and discuss in detail the following five questions. Each question should take you approximately thirty minutes, more or less.

- *When did you initially notice that your sexual desire was no longer as strong as it was before?* Please don't say that you are not quite sure. Everyone, with enough thought, can almost pinpoint precisely when desire began to drop. If you are still not sure, the next question may help.

- *Was there a life-changing event, situation, or trauma that occurred around the time that you no longer felt like having sex?* I am willing to bet that there was something that changed. Maybe your partner ignored you at a party. Or, a loved one died. Or, you changed jobs. Or, you moved to a new location. Or, there was a birth or an adoption of a child. Or, you began taking care of an elderly parent. Or, your adult child left the family system. The examples are endless. Nonetheless, figure out exactly what altered that could account for your change in sexual desire.

- *Tell your partner what he or she is doing, or not doing, that could possibly turn your sex centers off.* Is there lack of communication, excitement, or romance in your relationship? Or, perhaps your partner is not your champion. This means he or she does not support or stick up for you in front of parents, in-laws, siblings, friends, or coworkers. Or, he or she constantly criticizes everything you do. Or, he or she isn't spending enough time with you. Or, your partner demands too much of your time. Or, he or she is too passive. Or, your partner is too aggressive or pushy. For example, your partner criticizes, withholds feelings, or is defensive. Or, he or she whines, sulks, speaks too loudly or softly, or expects you to read his or her mind during a conversation. Does your partner ignore you? Is he or she too dependent on you? Does he or she lack empathy? You get the picture. Choose carefully; only discuss the ones that actually throw cold water on your sex drive.

- *Does your partner have any habits that you consider unpleasant or annoying?* There are zillions of habits. For example, he leaves the toilet seat up, she chews with her mouth open, he does not brush his teeth before kissing you, does not take a shower before lovemaking, leaves the milk out, is a clean freak, is messy, is a sloppy dresser, is late for engagements, slurps her coffee, watches TV too much, or does not turn the lights off before going to bed. The list is endless. We all have habits that annoy our partners that we are totally unaware of. Only address the habits that make you want to jump out of your shoes.

Now, relax and think about the information you and your partner just gathered. Don't try to resolve anything. For now, give yourself time to process, and then get some rest.

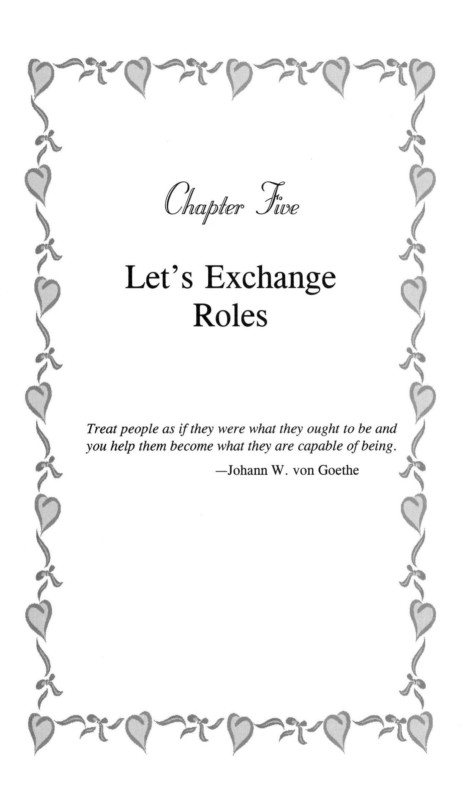

Chapter Five

Let's Exchange Roles

*Treat people as if they were what they ought to be and
you help them become what they are capable of being.*

—Johann W. von Goethe

This chapter was written to help you conceptualize the obstacles to sexual desire, as explained in the last chapter. I'm also going to throw in things we haven't addressed yet so you can begin to identify other factors that interfere with a sexual relationship.

Now, I'm going to ask you and your partner to read through the following scenario involving Jan and Jeff. See if you can identify the obstacles either learned from the last chapter or not yet discussed that interfere with their sexual desire. I believe that if you detach yourselves from personal feelings, you can clearly identify these obstacles that this couple, as well as yourselves, may face, without the filter of subjective emotion. Are you ready to vicariously assume the role of therapist? This will be fun.

Jan and Jeff

Jan and Jeff have been married for two years and have no children. Jan requested therapy because her desire for sex has gone down the tubes, and she's afraid it means she no longer loves her husband. As with most people who lose their desire, she had no idea of the obstacles causing her to turn off sexually.

They automatically slid into a traditional relationship where she stayed home and he went to work. During the week, Jan cleaned the house, did their laundry, cooked meals, ironed their clothes, and maintained the home while Jeff worked outside the home as a private investigator.

Each Saturday, Jeff would hang out with his buddies, and Jan would play cards with her girlfriends. They spent Sundays together with his parents.

After one year of staying home, Jan began to feel bored and sought employment as a hostess at a local restaurant. She loved her job and the people with whom she worked. She worked a thirty-hour week, but did not make much money. Jeff began to complain that the house was cluttered, his clothes were dirty, and he missed having dinner waiting for him when he came home from work. Jan tried to keep up with what she considered her wifely chores, but to no avail. She was just too exhausted when she came home from work. Although she asked Jeff for help, he felt she was responsible for the housework.

Since Jeff felt her income made little difference financially, he demanded that she quit her job. Although she loved her job, she complied. She was, however, both furious and embarrassed that he viewed her job as worthless.

Shortly afterwards, Jan found herself doing small things to irritate Jeff. She violated every pet peeve he had ever shared with her. She would leave dirty sponges in the sink, leave her shoes in the middle of their closet, over-starch his shirts, and leave both seats up on the toilet, which would make her laugh her head off when she'd hear a splash in the middle of the night. You get the picture. When Jeff accused her of doing these things intentionally, she would smile and say in a childlike voice, "No, I swear I'm not doing these things to make you angry."

What happened next should not surprise you. Jan began to reject Jeff's requests for sex. Initially, she turned him down occasionally; however, it quickly developed into a drop in desire. Even when she wanted to make love, she could not seem to get herself in the mood no matter how hard she tried. Jeff, in turn, felt rejected and unloved. He accused Jan of having an affair, which led to an ugly fight. This was the first serious argument of their marriage. That's when they called me for help.

When they arrived for their session, they sat down as far away from one another as possible. Neither even looked at each other. Here is a short excerpt of their initial session.

Therapist: What brings the two of you in today?

Jeff: *(in an angry voice)* I'll cut to the chase. We haven't had sex for months. No matter what I do, she just does not respond. I'm sick of it and I think the ice princess is either having an affair or wants a divorce. So, if that's what she wants, she can have it. If she thinks someone else will do it for her, then she's free to leave. I caught her flirting with my friend a few times; maybe she thinks he could turn her on. I'm a man, and all men need sex. If she doesn't give it to me, I'll find someone who will.

Jan: *(in a soft, whiney voice)* Please Jeff, don't threaten me. I'm not having an affair and I don't want a divorce. You are just an idiot. We wouldn't be here if I wanted a divorce. I don't know what's wrong. I used to love sex, and now I can't stand the thought of it. I'm just not excited about making love anymore. I don't know what's wrong with me. *(She burst into tears.)* I don't know what you're talking about when you said I was flirting with your stupid friends. You are the one who flirts with anything under the sun.

Jeff: *(furious)* Stop crying and grow up. The reason you're not excited about making love is that you're boring. You only know one position, and it's the same old thing night after night. Of course, that was when we even had sex. I haven't seen action in two months. You can't even get off without taking forever.

Jan: *(angry, but in her whiney voice)* Oh? You really think that I even get off? I don't think so. You are the one who's boring. Maybe if you got a book you'd know what to do and I would be excited. Instead, we do the same thing over and over.

Jeff: No sweetheart, you should read some books. You are the one with the problem.

Jan: The problem is my life. It's boring. You go to work, come home, eat dinner, want sex, and go to sleep. I'm home all day acting like a slave. I hate my life.

Jeff: If your life is so bad, leave. Just leave! *(Jeff jumped up off the couch and stormed out of the office. At this point Jan was laughing hysterically.)*

Jeff returned and took his place on the couch.

Jeff: Sorry Doc, but she makes me so mad, I can't see straight. *(looking at Jan)* You're an idiot, I swear. Don't you know how much I love you? The only reason I work so many hours is for you. I want us to have a nice home someday.

Jan: *(speaking in a whisper)* I know you work hard, Jeff. I love you too. That's why we're here. I don't know what's wrong with me.

Isn't this the most emotionally and verbally abusive couple you have ever encountered? I rarely see couples behave this horribly. I did, however, choose them to illustrate the worst-case scenario.

Okay, it's your turn. What would you do if you were their therapist? They certainly had their work cut out for them. It took over a year in therapy for them to resolve their issues enough to begin to lift sexual desire. You'll be happy to learn that they did develop power and reciprocity, and Jan's desire was restored.

Now, I'd like you and your partner to point out the obstacles that you feel turned off Jan's sex centers. A hint: Although it's Jan's sex centers that are turned off, Jeff is contributing greatly to her hypoactive sexual desire disorder. Take a few minutes to think about it, then continue reading for the answers.

Inequality within the Relationship

Did you guess it? Yes, this was the first obstacle that had to be removed. Jeff was controlling the marriage. He honestly felt that he had the right to force Jan to remain at home and take care of his needs. Jan, in turn, felt that it was her wifely duty to give in to his demands.

Jan resented her situation and began to engage in passive-aggressive behaviors; this made her feel like she had some control. In addition, she had total control regarding whether or not they would have sex. Jeff had no say in the matter. After weeks of refusing sex, she managed to temporarily turn off her sex centers, which then led to a sexual desire disorder.

Flirtatious Behavior

They each accused the other of being flirtatious. Yet, neither of them explored the reasons behind these accusations. If flirting did exist, they needed to take responsibility for this behavior, apologize to the other, and remove it permanently from their relationship.

Inability to Discuss Sexual Issues

Although they were both aware that sex was getting boring, they never engaged in an honest and frank sexual discussion. Instead, they complained and demeaned one another. This brings us to the next obstacle.

Ineffective Communication Skills

Neither actively listened to the other. Jeff's voice intonation was loud and threatening, and Jan's was whiney and childlike. They constantly interrupted each other and invalidated the other's position. They called each other demeaning names like "idiot" and "ice princess." Their eye contact was minimal.

They were defensive and blaming. Neither took responsibility for their own feelings, frequently using *you are* messages instead of *I feel* messages. There was zero empathy; and you got the feeling that neither felt love for the other. In addition, they used mind reading. Jeff thought that Jan wanted a divorce, which was something she totally denied.

This couple had the worst communication skills I had ever witnessed during all my years as a therapist.

An Intimate Boundary Was Missing

It is clear that their boundary was weak, almost to the point of disengagement. They sat as far apart from one another as they possibly could during their initial session.

Although they verbally professed their love for one another, they certainly didn't show love by their disrespectful actions.

They disengaged socially, which was manifested by Jeff being with his friends on Saturday and Jill playing cards with her friends. In addition, they spent every Sunday with his parents instead of one another. Again, I'm certainly not saying that there is something wrong with spending time with friends or family. For this couple, however, the weekends were the only time they had to be alone. They needed to take an occasional weekend for themselves.

They didn't quite fit the definition of a disengaged couple, because they were aware that their relationship wasn't working and were connected enough to seek help.

Lack of Connected Conversations

To be able to engage in connected conversations, intimacy, respect, and passion are needed. Obviously, neither authentically revealed their thoughts or feelings. The manner in which they spoke to each other was appallingly disrespectful. And they certainly didn't know how to have positive and passionate arguments. Instead, they engaged in ugly fights.

Individual Power Was Nonexistent

Jeff behaved like a controlling bully, which automatically rendered him powerless. His need to control caused him to scream and yell to get his own way. It's the adult version of a temper tantrum. Did Jan listen to his point of view when he behaved like such a child? She did not. As a matter of fact, she burst out laughing when he stormed out of the office. Did Jan possess power? No, she did not. She rendered herself powerless when she allowed Jeff to control her actions. Did Jeff listen to Jan's point of view? No, who would listen to someone whine and speak like a child? How could Jeff possibly take her concerns seriously? In addition, she did not address her complaints to Jeff directly, instead she used passive-aggressive behavior. Does this game playing ever work? Never.

Power Reciprocity

Do you think that Jan empowered Jeff, and vice versa? No, they did not. How on earth could they empower one another if neither one of them possessed a grain of individual power themselves. Individual power is essential for reciprocity to exist. As you will soon discover, individual power and power reciprocity have to be present first for sexual desire to be present. There are absolutely no exceptions to this rule.

I have a great deal of admiration for couples like Jan and Jeff. They had the courage to work so hard at saving their relationship. Surprisingly, this was a couple totally committed to resolving many conflicts within their relationship, and they were successful at ameliorating their sexual desire disorder.

I hope you gained some insight into your own unique obstacles. The next chapter briefly outlines physiologic obstacles that are mainly individual issues.

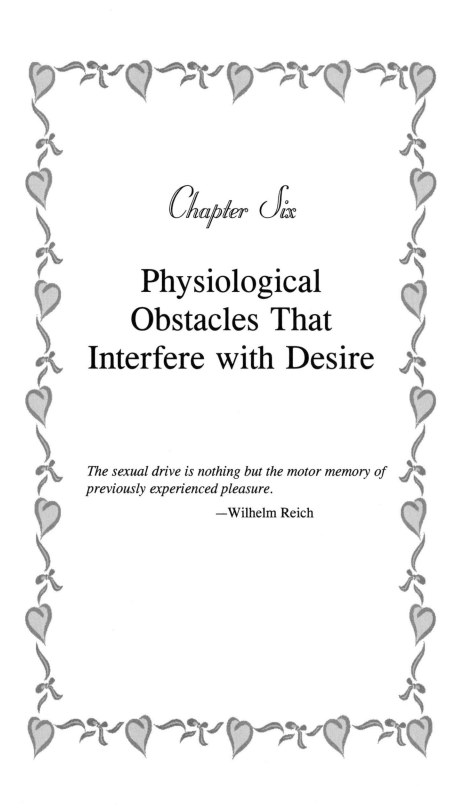

Chapter Six

Physiological Obstacles That Interfere with Desire

The sexual drive is nothing but the motor memory of previously experienced pleasure.

—Wilhelm Reich

While the focus of this book is on interrelationship issues, I would be remiss, if I didn't briefly address the individual ones as well. Individual obstacles can be psychological, pharmacological, hormonal, or medical in nature. Once these obstacles are addressed, this book will be extremely useful regarding your sexual relationship. Although there are too many individual obstacles to mention I have included the more common ones.

Alcohol and Substance Abuse

Let's start with some facts about drugs. In our society, drugs, including alcohol, have long been associated with removing sexual inhibitions and hence making sexual activities more pleasurable. The reason is that these substances can have an effect on the dopamine receptors within the brain, which can cause euphoric feelings and decrease sexual inhibition. However, any individual who chronically abuses alcohol or other substances over time can experience hypoactive sexual desire disorder. Overuse of alcohol, in fact, profoundly depresses the central nervous system, and that can actually anesthetize sexual feelings. Take heart, if you are abusing drugs or alcohol, there are many community support groups and treatment centers that can help you. All you have to do is reach out.

Depression

Depression is manifested by sadness, anxiety, helplessness, hopelessness, pessimism, difficulty concentrating or making decisions, fatigue, irritability, low self-esteem, eating or sleeping changes, loss of interest or pleasure in activities that you once enjoyed (including sex), and suicidal thoughts. Depression also causes people to have negative thoughts about themselves. Negative thoughts cause powerlessness. Without power, sexual desire is nonexistent.

Depression has variable degrees of severity, which may or may not require medication. If you do, however, take antidepressant medication, you need to know that some of the most widely prescribed antidepressants have sexual side effects that can decrease sexual desire. A common side effect of Selective Serotonin Reuptake Inhibitors (SSRI) is a drop in libido. If you are taking one of the SSRIs, you may or may not experience this side effect. Wellbutrin and Deseryl, on the other hand, have been known to increase sexual desire while decreasing the depression. It is worth discussing with your physician the sexual side effects of any medication you are taking. However, if a person is depressed, the immediate priority is to lift depression. Depression is highly treatable, usually with good results. Once the depression is lifted, you can restore your sex life as it was prior to the onset of depression.

An Abnormal Hormonal Level

As mentioned, testosterone is a necessary hormone to keep sexual desire healthy. If you or your partner's level is below normal, your physician can prescribe appropriate amounts of this androgen. I do, however, want to remind you again that increasing your testosterone level is worthless, and sometimes dangerous, if your levels are normal. I rarely have seen a man or woman whose testosterone level, when tested, was found to be below normal levels. Many are disappointed when they hear this news, because they secretly hope that they can pop a magic pill and instantly increase desire. Sorry, nothing is that simple.

Although the hormone estrogen has zero effect on sexual desire, it is important to female lubrication. If there is a lack of estrogen, due to a hysterectomy, menopause, or chemotherapy, sexual intercourse will be downright painful if the female is not lubricated. You can bet that if intercourse is painful, the result will be a desire disorder. Ask your gynecologist for recommendations regarding hormone replacement therapy especially in light of a recent research study addressing the dangerous risk factors attached to HRT. A possible alternative could be the use of creams, ointments, or an over-the-counter lubricant (K-Y Jelly).

If a male's prolactin hormone level is high, his libido will drop quickly to zero. This condition is known as hyper-prolactinemia, which is a serious, but very rare, condition that needs to be addressed by a physician immediately.

Poor Physical Health

Suffering from poor physical health due to a medical condition can certainly interfere with your sex centers. After all, I cannot think of anyone who would want to engage in any activity, including sex, if they just don't feel well. In addition, specific disorders like diabetes affect sexual performance, and such concerns could affect sexual desire. I do, however, suggest that you continue to read this book so you will be well prepared once your health improves.

The Effects of Aging

I have good news for you. The pleasure of sexuality does not end until the day we die! As we age, however, our bodies do go through certain physiologic changes that affect sexual desire. For example, most people's eyesight is fine when they are young. They cannot even imagine what life would be like with poor eyesight, because they take their sight for granted, believing it will never change. As people age, they often notice that they have more and more difficulty reading and driving at night. Finally, they realize they need to obtain corrective lenses.

It's a similar situation with sexuality. People, especially men, have a hard time imagining that their sexual drive will someday change. We have to adapt to changes by maintaining a positive attitude and taking whatever steps necessary to enhance what we have at any given time. Plus, we have to maintain positive attitudes about ourselves as we age. I want to remind you that the following information is variable and is only to be used as a guideline. Each person is different.

Men and Aging

Let's take a look at the typical changes men go through during the aging process. During adolescence, males experience intensity in their sexual desire. They are preoccupied with thoughts of sex, and it takes very little provocation to achieve a firm erection. Orgasms are plentiful, either with a partner or through masturbation, and ejaculation is forceful. Actually, eight orgasms per day are not all that unusual for an adolescent. Their intensity is only lessened by a small degree into the twenties.

During their thirties, men continue to be highly sexual, and erection continues to be easy to obtain. However, they are satisfied with one orgasm per day. Sexual desire is high during this phase if the male is in good health and does not abuse drugs or alcohol.

During their forties and fifties, men's sexual sensation will begin to change. Achieving an erect penis is not as easy to come by as it was during the earlier phases. In other words, men do not spring into action by a sexy thought or by the sight of their lover; they need much more hands-on stimulation. They are now satisfied with one or two orgasms per week; however, ejaculation is not as forceful. Men become quite concerned because they are aware that their once high libido is lessened, even though the sexual experience continues to remain pleasurable.

There are several noted theorists who have stated that perhaps men experience a male menopause climacteric (Mulligan and Moss 1991) because sexual desire decreases so drastically. This is due to the fact that the testes stop producing as much testosterone as they did earlier. Men experience symptoms similar to those that women exhibit during menopause, which can include irritability, feeling blue, developing a negative body image, and loss of physical strength. They begin to become aware of the fact that they are no longer the sexually virile male of their youth. I am sure you have all heard about some of the irrational decisions that are made during this period to boost the male ego. For example, buying a red sports car and becoming sexually involved with a much younger woman are two of the most common symptoms of so-called male climacteric.

By the time the male reaches about sixty, sexual desire drops off considerably. However, with enough physical stimulation, an erection can be achieved. When he has an orgasm, ejaculation is less forceful. So what? He and his partner can still enjoy lovemaking. Remember, the sexual experience is so much more than intercourse. It has been well documented that men in their nineties can enjoy sex twice a week. If men enjoyed sex in younger years, they will continue to enjoy sex during the later years.

I have, however, seen signs of aging in a male turn into a serious obstacle. He may view his hair loss, wrinkles, and loss of physical strength as a loss of power. A looming retirement may have a negative effect as well. Power, however, has nothing at all to do with wrinkles, hair loss, or a limited income. If the male can maintain his power, sexual desire will remain intact.

Women and Aging

For women, it is a different story. During adolescence, women are typically less interested in being sexually active than they are in gaining intimacy. Actually, they are more interested in the idea of having what they consider an "intimate relationship." Often, sex is the exchange that young women make for intimacy. Compared to young men, fewer young women have the urge to masturbate. They do, however, have an active fantasy life. In their late twenties, most females are just beginning to enjoy their sexuality. They become more assertive, secure, and take charge of their own sexuality.

By the time a woman is in her mid to late thirties, she is at her sexual peak. She masturbates frequently, lubricates easily, often has multiple orgasms, has a rich sexual fantasy life, and is more demanding of having a partner with sexual skills.

During their forties and fifties, most women are beginning or are in the throes of menopause. Vaginal lubrication can be problematic. Without adequate lubrication, sexual intercourse can be downright painful. Unlike men, the woman's clitoral sensitivity and orgasms are not affected in this age group. As a matter of fact, studies show that a woman's orgasms increase with each decade and continue right through her nineties. Sexual desire continues to be normal unless her testosterone level drops below a normal level.

By age sixty, women continue to be multiorgasmic; however, the intensity of orgasm is lessened. So what? They are still pretty great! As with men, if women have enjoyed sex in the past, they will continue to enjoy sex into their nineties.

Yes, we'll all get to be elderly, if we're lucky. If we remain in good physical health and view ourselves in a positive light, sexual activities will continue to be pleasurable and gratifying. As with males, the major obstacle is having a negative attitude about getting older. I cannot emphasize enough the advantage of having a good attitude. With a good attitude, we continue to have positive thoughts about ourselves.

It's been well documented that with age, we become less sexually inhibited, which translates into enjoying better sex. After sixty, one small change a couple can make is to have sex in the morning, instead of at night. That way you have both had a good night's sleep.

Come on now, you don't need a break. This was an easy chapter to get through. The next chapter is extremely fun. It does, however, require work.

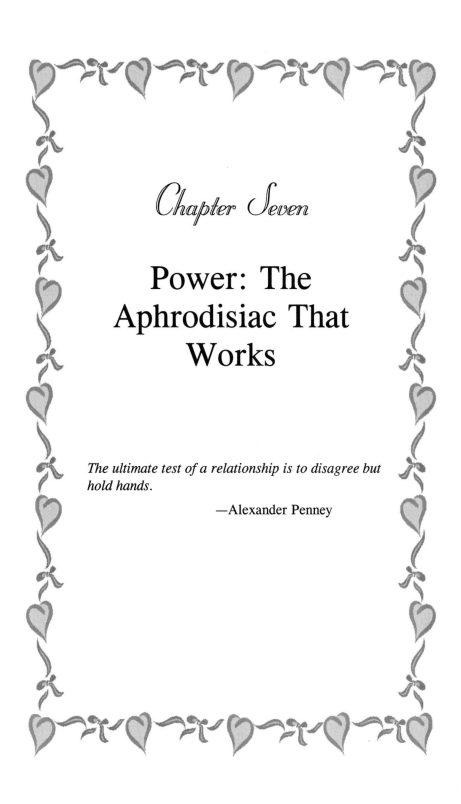

Chapter Seven

Power: The Aphrodisiac That Works

The ultimate test of a relationship is to disagree but hold hands.

—Alexander Penney

Throughout history, humankind has been in search of the magic bullet that creates sexual desire. We have tried everything from ground-up beetles, seaweed, herbs, love potions, and street drugs to alcohol, salves, certain foods, injections, and pills. The truth is that few of these so-called aphrodisiacs actually work and worse yet, some can cause harm or death. That is why I am delighted to announce that there is an aphrodisiac that is not only safe, it actually works. And the best news is that you need look no further than yourself to find it. What is it? I am sure by now you know because I've been alluding to it throughout the previous chapters; the answer is power. Let's examine the concept of power.

Understanding Power

Forget everything you ever knew or thought you knew about what power is. In relationships, power takes on a whole new meaning. In ordinary language, we use the word *power* in several different ways. Often we speak of power in terms of physical ability, as in the strength or force of a boxer's punch. Within a political context, power can mean having the ability to rule, govern, or control. When we talk of power in a psychological context, to have power over someone can mean manipulating that person for our own gain. None of these connotations of power relate to, or work for, you and your relationship. There are two types of power, genuine and toxic power. Let's briefly distinguish between the two.

Genuine Power

The concept of genuine power means possessing a quality that most people find influential, impressive, convincing, and sexy. It is about the ability to produce a positive effect on yourself as well as others. Genuine power is about discovering who you really are, what you stand for, and how you are going to use your voice to make something positive happen.

How Do We Recognize Genuine Power in Others?

You know when you are in the presence of individuals who are genuinely powerful, because empowering others seems to come naturally. They automatically empower everyone in their space. When they speak, we listen. And when we speak, they listen. These are the people who have discovered contentment and joy in their lives. They never try to make another person feel less important than they are. They are the individuals who love their partners as much as they love themselves and make their relationship a top priority. These are the individuals who share their power, joy, and contentment with others.

Genuine power earns its name, because it is never dependent on making others feel small. In fact, the more those with genuine power share their power with others, the more that power comes back to them, and the more powerful they feel. People with genuine power feel great about themselves. People who possess genuine power are sexy.

Unfortunately, the word power often has a negative connotation in our language as well.

Toxic Power

Toxic power is also about being influential, impressive, and convincing, but the difference is these individuals use their power to make something negative happen.

How Do We Recognize Those with Toxic Power?

Those with toxic power use their voice, opinions, influence, persuasion, sexuality, and authority to manipulate, dominate, and control others. This form of power is like a poisonous gas that slowly depletes the integrity of other individuals.

Unfortunately, most of us know people who fit this description. Perhaps this person was your teacher, your doctor, a boss, a family member, or a significant other. These individuals lack integrity, values, and character. They abuse their individual power to get their own needs met, regardless of the negative ramifications it may cause to others. They use their charm, intelligence, and persuasion to exploit others' trusting natures, vulnerabilities, or weaknesses.

Toxic power is feeble, for it is insecurity based; toxic individuals can only feel powerful by making others feel weak and vulnerable. For this reason, toxic power is one-sided and unequal; it is never reciprocated.

If you have ever felt attracted to someone who had toxic power, it was undoubtedly at a time when you yourself felt powerless. The reason you found this person attractive was because he or she had what you mistakenly perceived as power. When we feel powerless, we fool ourselves into believing that being around a powerful person will make us feel powerful as well. However, a person with toxic power is never interested in sharing it. On the other hand, when we develop a strong sense of individual power, our need to be around others with toxic power disappears.

Let's move on to something amazingly positive. This will be a turning point in your sexual desire. You will be able to open up your sex centers as well as your partner's. All you have to do is begin to understand your own sense of power.

Understanding Your Own Individual Power

It is vitally important to realize that power is not just reserved for the fortunate few. Every person on the face of this planet is born with power; we only just forget sometimes that it is there inside us for the asking. You will soon learn how to tap into this power.

If you were lucky enough to have had parents who empowered you as a child, then you likely grew up to be a powerful adult. Unfortunately, a lot of people did not have this type of parenting. Most of us grew up hearing messages like, "Children should be seen and not heard," or "Do what I say, not what I do." This does not mean that your parents did not love you. It just means that they did not develop the best parenting skills. Nonetheless, if you learned as a child that your opinions did not matter, you could have developed into someone who feels powerless. The good news is that it is never too late to develop the traits needed for power and power reciprocity.

Power begins inside of you. You have to feel great about who you are and what you stand for. Power is an active attribute; it is something that you manifest through your words and actions. In other words, if you have powerful thoughts or ideas but never share these thoughts or ideas with another person, they mean nothing. They have to be shared through your words and actions. Power resides in the way others listen to you and are influenced and persuaded by what you have to say.

Power reciprocity is using your own individual power to empower your partner, while your partner will use his or her own individual power to empower you. In other words, whatever you give your partner will be returned in kind, and vice versa.

Exercise: Power Revealed

Power reveals itself through internal beliefs and external actions. I'd like you and your partner to go through the following statements and determine what components you possess or what may be temporarily missing. Remember, all you have to do is tap into what already exists in you. Relax; you and your partner will learn exactly how to develop individual power in the next chapter. For now, quickly go through these statements.

- You are powerful when you are aware of who you are and what you stand for.

- You are powerful when you can state your views in a clear, concise, and persuasive manner.

- You are powerful when you have a choice in every decision you make.

- You are powerful when you are emotionally and financially independent.

- You are powerful when you have the courage to do anything you set your mind to do.

- You are powerful when you have the bravery to share your personal opinions and beliefs with your partner.

- You are powerful when you have the courage to convince, influence, and persuade your partner.

- You are powerful when you have the capacity to provide direction to your partner.

- You are powerful when you know your values and make a stand to defend these values.

- You are powerful when you are being authentic.

- You are powerful when you have integrity, that is, being true to your word.

The Prerequisites of Power Reciprocity

With power comes responsibility. Power is not something to wield over your partner; it is something to be shared. This is the essence of power reciprocity, and this is what keeps sexual desire alive in your relationship.

Exercise: Exchanging Power

Determine whether you or your partner currently has an understanding of how to reciprocate power. If you do, I would be shocked! Most people don't have the foggiest idea as to how to exchange power. I, for one, had to learn how to develop this amazing skill. You will soon discover exactly how to do it. For now, take yourselves through this brief exercise to learn the basics of power reciprocity.

Power reciprocity requires:

- That you understand your own feelings and motivations.

- That you understand your partner's feelings and motivations. The more you know about your partner, the better you can determine what you could do or say to help your partner feel more powerful.

- That you listen carefully to what your partner says, and you expect the same courtesy.

- That you listen to your partner, even if he or she has different opinions, and you expect your partner to do the same.

- That you connect to your partner on an emotional level when you communicate, and you insist that your partner connect to you. Power reciprocity demands a profound level of communication.

How Does Power Affect the Sex Centers?

At times, negative thoughts, feelings, and circumstances can short-circuit your sense of individual power and thus your desire for sex. I will give you an example of when my own individual power was short-circuited. I have been doing media work for the past fourteen years. I am used to being in front of the TV cameras. I love sharing my knowledge with thousands of viewers, and I enjoy the limelight. I very seldom get anxious, and I arm myself with the latest possible research, regarding the topic of the show. Plus, I consider myself to be an extremely powerful woman who is not afraid to speak her mind and get others to listen. Being a therapist has helped me to be an interested listener as well.

About two years ago, I was invited to appear on a local TV show to discuss, "Is flirting harmless?" I prepared myself and had plenty to say about the topic, as you already know. I arrived at the station ready to go, but five minutes before the show, the producer raced out to greet me, totally out of breath.

She said, "Dr. Cervenka, there has just been a news release regarding a horrible tragedy involving several suicides. All of these people were involved in a cult and the cult leader called for the suicides of his members. And then he killed himself. So, instead of doing the show we planned, we need you to discuss how cult leaders control their members."

I was dumbstruck. "Cults?" I said. "I don't know anything about cults! I can't do this!"

The producer laughed and said, "Stop worrying, you'll do just fine." And so the show began. With the TV camera pointed at me and the lights blazing, the host of the show asked me the first question, then the second, then the third, and on and on. It was the longest show of my life. I had zero research-based information, which is something that I rely on to answer questions professionally. But in this situation, I was forced to answer using my own personal opinions. I strongly believe that no professional should ever use his or her own personal opinions in place of well-founded research or clinical experience when asked for expert advice. Personal opinions are for connected conversations, not for disseminating information to the public. With each answer, I could feel my power drain from my spirit. I did, however, alert the public that my answers were personal opinions.

After the program was over, the producer told me that everyone thought the show was great. I, however, knew that I had used my own personal opinions and not science. On my drive home, I kept thinking, "I can't believe I answered those questions with my own opinions. That was stupid and unprofessional."

By the time I pulled in my driveway, I felt about as powerful as a gnat. My husband, who is my greatest champion, thought the interview was great and welcomed me home by having a beautiful candlelit dinner. After dinner, he expressed that he felt like making love, but I certainly did not. When you feel powerless, you do not feel too sexy. As a matter of fact, I felt like an ineffectual lump of lard.

Sensing my mood, my husband told me that there are times when personal opinions are just as important as research-based information. He also added that he found my opinions informative and useful.

"They were?" I said.

"You always do the best you can," he said, "and that is what is important. You were able to do something that most people, including myself, could not do. I am proud of you."

Because I view my husband as powerful and respect his opinions, I felt my own power rushing back. He had used his power (getting me to listen to his point of view) to help me feel my individual power again. And guess what? Feeling powerful is an internal sexual turn-on. And viewing your partner as powerful is an external turn-on. Because of this exchange of power, which is what power reciprocity is all about, I was able to quickly turn on my brain's sex centers and we experienced fireworks in the bedroom that evening.

The point of this story is this: you cannot turn on your brain's sex centers unless power is present within yourself as well as your partner and is exchanged equally within your relationship. When you have these components of power, you and your partner will also experience fireworks in the bedroom, because you will have restored sexual desire. Remember, you cannot have great sex unless you have sexual desire in the first place. And to have sexual desire, you need individual power and power reciprocity.

If my husband did not possess individual power in my eyes, the outcome of this scenario could have turned out to be quite different. What if, for example, he was envious of my being on TV? What if he was insecure and needed to compete with me? What if he did not know how to emotionally connect with me in a conversation? What if he was not my champion? What if he lacked the skills to empower me?

In any one of these scenarios, he could have said, "Oh well, there will be other shows"—an emotionally disconnected approach that would ignore my feelings rather than convince me to feel differently. Or, "I cannot believe you even went on that show without knowing what you were talking about"—participating in my own self-punishment, which would perpetuate my feelings of powerlessness. Or, "Maybe you should stop doing media work"—letting me know I was a failure in his eyes, which would also reinforce my feelings of powerlessness. Or, "Come on honey, I will take your mind off of your embarrassment, let's go in the bedroom"—completely skipping a step; namely, doing his best to empower me so that I would feel desire for sex.

In any of these cases, I would have been temporarily stuck with those feelings of powerlessness, and my sex centers would have remained shut down until I regained my power on my own. Plus, I would have had feelings of resentment and contempt toward him. Those feelings are sex extinguishers. Thank goodness I am married to a man who is powerful in his own right and therefore does not see my individual power as a threat.

Because my husband and I continually empower each other, our sexual desire remains high after twenty-three years together. So as you can see, it's not enough that you and your partner possess individual power; it's essential to have reciprocal power.

Although it is crucial that we do what we can to empower our partner and are open to letting our partner empower us, it is also important that we take personal responsibility for restoring our own individual sense of power. In this situation, let's take a look at what led to my feelings of powerlessness.

First of all, I took myself a bit too seriously. After all, the planet was not hanging on every word I uttered. That was not about power at all; that was arrogance. If I had actually tapped into my true power, I would have told myself, "I will do my best. I will state my opinions clearly and the world will not end if I do not have all the answers."

Once You Achieve Power, Is It a Constant?

No. In any relationship, individual power and power reciprocity can transform into wimpiness and powerless reciprocity. The good news is that you can always turn around the situation and get back into a place of power.

To explain this process, let's say that you and your partner are engaged in an intimate conversation that you are both enjoying. Your positive communication, smiling face, and laughter will explicitly influence your partner's mood. In turn, your partner's positive communication, smiles, and laughter will have an explicit effect on your mood as well. Do you see the reciprocity in this situation? It's like a circle that has no end. You say something positive, he reacts to your positive statements, and you in turn react to his positive statements, and on and on. At this point, each of you is offering something powerful to the conversation.

This circular process will continue unless something negative is said, implied, or misunderstood to change this mood from positive to negative. It does not matter who voiced the negative or misunderstood statement. This statement, whether intended or not, can affect your partner's mood, which will elicit a negative response from your partner, and affect your mood as well. In turn, your negative mood will have an effect on him or her. You are now engaged in powerless reciprocity. As you can see, reciprocity has no end, because it goes round and round. If either of you feels powerless or diminished by what the other has said, your desire for sexual contact will disappear.

At this point, one or both of you has to transform this powerless reciprocity by acting powerfully. For example, you could say, "I did not like what you said. What exactly did you mean by that statement? I would like to resolve this right now." If you know how to have healthy arguments, you will be able to return to your powerful positions and restore power reciprocity.

I experienced this situation one night when I excitedly told my husband of a theory I created regarding relationships. As I spoke, I noticed he was laughing, which I perceived as, *He must think that my theory is idiotic.* Furious, I sulked and stopped talking for a few minutes until I regained my power. If power reciprocity was missing in our relationship, the entire conversation could have broken down. I could have assumed that my perception was the truth and gone to bed angry and hurt. Thank goodness power was alive and well in both of us that evening.

I confronted him and said, "Why are you laughing at me?"

He said, "I am not laughing at you at all. I am laughing because I am excited for you. I have never met anyone before who invented a theory about relationships."

Power reciprocity could have short-circuited if I had not made the choice to confront him with my perception of his laughter. It is always a choice whether reciprocity will be powerful or powerless.

Power is the best mental aphrodisiac known to mankind. It's extremely sexy. Now, relax and remember that power lives within you. After you are both rested, we are going to take a look at the antithesis of power. What is it? Turn the page to find out.

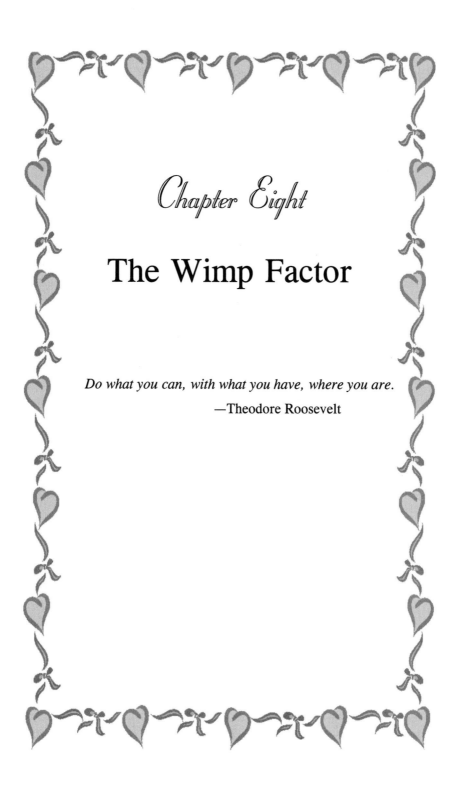

Chapter Eight

The Wimp Factor

Do what you can, with what you have, where you are.
—Theodore Roosevelt

As you are now aware, physical appearance was the initial attraction that triggered sexual desire; however, power and power reciprocity are what support that sexual attraction throughout the lifetime of a relationship.

Survey Results

Based on a survey I conducted with hundreds of men and women regarding attributes that are sexually desirable, a top priority was a partner they perceived as powerful. I asked heterosexual men and women what they considered to be the sexiest component that they subscribed to the opposite sex. I also asked gay men and lesbians to answer this question with the same sex in mind. The following will examine the results of the survey.

What Do Men Consider Sexy?

Excluding physical appearance, most men stated that the women they consider sexy possess self-confidence, are financially and emotionally independent, make decisions on their own, are comfortable with confrontation, and can openly discuss issues. In other words, men described women who were powerful.

What Do Women Consider to Be Sexually Desirable?

Excluding physical appearance, most women consider men who are powerful to be sexy. This was described as the guys who took charge, were decisive, could not be controlled, were forceful in their opinions, possessed high self-esteem, had the ability to emotionally connect, and would be their champion.

Are Gays and Lesbians Any Different in What They Perceive to Be Sexy?

No, there is absolutely no difference at all. The only difference between gay and straight is sexual preference. Gays and lesbians also ranked power as the number one turn-on. Men and women, gay or straight, agreed that being with someone who fits the stereotype of what society considers physically attractive was not as important as being with someone they perceived as powerful.

How Do Women Describe Non-Sexy Men?

In the same survey these same individuals were asked to use one word describing someone who had little or no sex appeal. Excluding physical appearance, most women chose the word "wimp." Women just don't view powerless men as sexy. When men were asked how they would feel if their partner called them a wimp, their answers were unanimous. "No man wants to be considered a wimp. It's the worst! Who wants to be viewed as impotent? It's the most emasculating word a woman could use." In other words, all men view this term as an attack to their masculinity. I can't say that I blame them.

How Do Men Describe a Non-Sexy Woman?

Men chose two words to describe a woman with little sex appeal, excluding physical appearance, "needy and dependent." All the women had a strong reaction to these words as well. "No woman wants to be considered needy and dependent. It describes someone who is subservient or childlike. I would hate it if my partner said that about me!" In other words, men described a female wimp.

As you can clearly see, the wimp factor, or powerlessness—a term I like better—is not a sexy attribute. In fact, it is impossible to experience sexual desire without possessing individual power and power reciprocity.

Don't All People Feel Powerless Once in a While?

Sure, most of us feel powerless at one time or another. The important thing is to develop the ability to recognize when we feel powerless and to take action to reclaim our power.

The first thing to do in transforming your state of powerlessness to one of power is to identify negative thoughts or feelings you have about yourself. Or, perhaps your partner said something hurtful—intentional or otherwise—that temporarily zapped your power. You need to have the courage to voice your concerns, even your hurts, with your partner. Remember my illustration of how I thought my husband was laughing at me?

Are There Situations That Can Trigger Powerlessness?

Yes, there are certain situations that can zap power. For example, what about the person who exudes power in the workplace but appears powerless at home? Or what about someone who loses power when in the presence of a parent? Years ago, I treated a couple experiencing a severe sexual desire disorder. The primary obstacle was an intrusive, paternal mother-in-law who lived with them. Once the obstacle was identified, the male was asked to confront his intrusive mother. Although he was extremely powerful in the workplace, he became powerless when in the presence of his mom. His partner viewed his powerlessness as wimpy, which turned off her sex centers. Once he was able to identify his powerlessness, he reclaimed it. This case study will be explained in more detail later in this chapter.

As the example illustrates, once you have identified that you are feeling powerless and the source of your powerlessness, you can reclaim your power. It's just a matter of finding your voice and having the courage to use it. You have a right to your own opinions, thoughts, and feelings, which gives you the right to voice them. If you feel like you do not have this right, you will become powerless, which is manifested by dependence, helplessness, and passivity.

Let's examine how powerlessness played itself out in a relationship where infidelity was the obstacle. A high profile college educator, Ginny, requested my help. Known in the community as a powerful woman, Ginny spoke her mind and others listened.

In her relationship, however, she was powerless. Her husband, Drake, constantly cheated on her. In addition, he had been rejecting her sexually for the past six months. Here is a short excerpt of our initial telephone conversation.

Therapist: Ginny, why do you think Drake is being unfaithful?

Ginny:	I don't know. I try to look good for him, I cook his favorite meals, I buy sexy nightgowns, but nothing seems to work. Instead, he looks for other women to have sex with. I wish I didn't love him so much so I could just end it.
Therapist:	Why are you blaming yourself for his infidelities?
Ginny:	Why else would he have sex with other women if there wasn't something wrong with me?
Therapist:	Have you confronted him about these affairs?
Ginny:	No. He doesn't know that I know about them. I'm afraid he'll leave me if I confront him with this.
Therapist:	So, what you are telling me is that you are willing to live with a man who constantly betrays, deceives, and disrespects you, and you are not going to confront him? Do you understand that your silence is a form of agreement?
Ginny:	I know what you're saying, but I just can't bring it up with him.
Therapist:	It looks to me like you have two choices. You can continue to live with this pain or you can begin to take steps to change your situation.
Ginny:	*(crying)* I know that, but I cannot confront him, I just can't. He might leave me if I do that. I love him so much. Look, all I need from you are suggestions that will get him sexually interested in me again.
Therapist:	Ginny, suggestions won't help; it's not your fault that he is making these choices. The fact is, your marriage isn't working. You have a right to express the disappointment and pain that his infidelities cause.
Ginny:	I know what you are saying, but right now I just can't. I called you because I thought you could help me become sexier so that my husband would become interested in me again.

Therapist: Ginny, becoming sexier is not the issue. Not having power is your problem. I suggest you and Drake enter couple therapy as soon as possible.

Ginny angrily refused my request that they deal with these issues in couple therapy. She simply did not want to "upset things."

As you can see, Ginny's powerlessness was selective. Professionally, she was powerful. She was considered impressive, persuasive, and influential. In her relationship, however, she was afraid of confronting her husband. In asking me to tell her how to become sexy, she had missed the point entirely. I knew that unless she voiced her opinions, thoughts, and feelings to her husband, she would remain powerless in her relationship. Trying to appear sexier doesn't translate into the development of her power. It just doesn't work that way. You have to have power to be sexy, not the other way around.

What happened next might surprise you. Two months after I spoke to Ginny, Drake phoned me requesting couple therapy. He told me that he had confessed to having two short affairs and was shocked to discover that Ginny knew of his infidelities. He explained that he did love his wife; however, he was no longer sexually attracted to her. Here is a brief excerpt from our phone conversation.

Therapist: Drake, I don't get it. If you love Ginny, then why are you rejecting her sexually and betraying her by sleeping with other women?

Drake: I wish I had the answer. I feel ashamed and guilty about my affairs, and I don't understand why I don't feel sexually attracted to Ginny anymore. When I first met Ginny, she was strong, independent, and sexy. It was love at first sight, and our sex life was great. But as soon as we got married, she totally changed. She became dependent and needy. Don't get me wrong; she's the sweetest and kindest woman I have ever met. But she's just too clingy. I feel suffocated. She leaves all the decisions to me, and she agrees with every little thing I say. I have never seen her angry about anything. It's like living with a saint. She counts on me for almost everything. She actually told me that she would feel dead if I left the relationship. When I told her about my two affairs, she told me that she already knew about them. She wasn't even angry, she just cried and said she didn't want to lose me. I'll tell you this, if she had cheated on me, I would have hit the roof.

Therapist: You are actually telling me that you are blaming Ginny for something you choose to do? Granted, her dependency is a sexual turnoff, but you could have discussed your feelings with her. You, and you alone, are totally responsible for leaving the marital boundary, not her.

Drake: I know, I shouldn't blame her for my no longer being sexually attracted to her. I love Ginny, she's wonderful, but sex is important to me. If I can't get back my desire, we'll probably get divorced.

Therapist: I did not say that Ginny isn't part of the problem. What I said is that she's not responsible for your decision to sleep with other women. You told me that she's turning you off by her dependency. That is the issue that we need to discuss. You both appear to love one another; it's way too soon to think about divorce. I want to make clear that your lack of sexual desire is not just *your* sexual problem; it's a relationship problem. Before I see the two of you, however, I suggest that you take total responsibility for your actions and sincerely apologize for your betrayals. It will not be easy, and you'll have to be able to talk at great length about this with her. She'll have a million questions that you'll have to honestly answer. Then, you have to promise her that no matter what, you will never cheat on her again. If you do not restore dignity to your relationship, then neither of you will be able to work on sexual desire issues.

Drake: Okay, but I'm scared to death. I'm disgusted with myself. I know I hurt her badly, and I wish I could take it all back.

By the time we reached our tenth couple session together, Ginny finally found her voice and was able to tell Drake that his affairs hurt her terribly. She finally expressed her anger and told him that she would never go through that type of humiliation again. As she released her anger, I began to see her transformation. I could see her power start to return as she dropped her angelic self and spoke with conviction.

Drake listened intently and promised that he would never seek sexual favors from other women again. Drake found his own voice and told Ginny how he had viewed her as powerless, which for him was a sexual turnoff. She agreed to give up her neediness and dependency and to voice her opinions. So far, they are doing great in therapy. Power and power reciprocity are being restored, and so is their sexual desire.

Often when we look at a situation in which there is infidelity, our own or someone else's, we assume that the person who is cheating has all the power and the person who is being betrayed has none. This isn't exactly the case. Drake's inability to tell Ginny that he was turned off by her neediness, dependency, and submissiveness rendered him powerless in his relationship. Essentially, he was every bit as powerless as his wife was. For Drake, his own powerlessness to express himself openly with Ginny, along with his perception of Ginny as weak, killed any sexual desire he had for her. However, he still wanted sexual release, so he sought it elsewhere. I say this not to excuse his behavior but to explain it. The affairs, rather than making him feel powerful, made him feel disgusted with himself.

But what about Ginny? On the surface, it might appear that Ginny's request for tips on getting her husband sexually interested in her meant that she had desire for him. It did not. It simply indicated her desperate need to manipulate him back into the relationship, a way of proving to herself that their marriage was okay again. It was a way of denying what was really wrong with their relationship, by choosing to believe that the other women must have something that she did not.

Power and Perception

Often in relationships couples find themselves faced with a dilemma in which one partner wants sex but the other one does not. If we take a closer look at these relationships, this one-sided desire for sex is all about an imbalance of perceived power. The key word is *perceived*. Inevitably, the person who desires sex sees their partner as powerful. Nevertheless, even if your partner sees you as powerful, you will not feel desire for your partner unless you also see yourself as powerful; and of course, you must see your partner as powerful too. Similarly, if you feel powerless and also see your partner as weak, you'll have a double dose of powerlessness that will destroy your desire; that is, until you restore a balance of perceived power to your relationship.

This complex dynamic of perceived power can best be explained in the following illustration. As you read this, I'd like you to pick out where power and reciprocity are missing. I'll call this couple Luke and Marlene. Luke was a forty-year-old, extremely successful, and much sought-after attorney. When Luke spoke, everyone listened. He was persuasive, impressive, and influential at work. Marlene was a thirty-eight-year-old pediatrician with a successful practice who was also considered powerful by her peers and patients.

The pair had been married for seventeen years when they first came to me for therapy. For the first fifteen years of their marriage, they were happy, intimate, and committed. During those years, they had enjoyed an active and passionate sex life. For the last two years, however, Marlene had lost all sexual desire for Luke. As a result, they made love every six or seven months, and their lovemaking was without any passion. Luke's desire for Marlene, however, had not diminished. What was interesting was that each claimed to perceive the other as powerful, and each viewed themselves as powerful as well. I knew, however, they both lacked individual power and perceived one another as powerless. Otherwise, a desire disorder wouldn't be present.

Just as I had asked you to pinpoint some change that took place around the time that desire left, I asked them to do the same. I wanted them to think about what might have occurred around two years ago that could account for Marlene's loss of desire. The couple struggled with this question for almost ten minutes, and finally Luke came up with the birth of their second child as a possible obstacle. I asked them to face each other and discuss how they felt this child was interfering with their sex life.

Luke: Maybe the kids are exhausting you. Maybe you just don't have enough energy to make love any more.

Marlene: I don't think having Johnny was any different than when we had Cindy. I don't think that the birth of Johnny or spending time with the kids has anything to do with it.

Therapist: So you don't feel having a second child had anything to do with your lack of sexual desire?

Marlene: No, not at all.

Therapist: Do you feel Luke might be doing something that contributes to your lack of desire?

[It took her three minutes to answer that question.]

Marlene:	I never looked at it that way. I thought it was something that I was doing. All I know is that I am just not sexually attracted to him like I used to be.
Therapist:	Face Luke and tell him what could he possibly be doing to turn you off.
Marlene:	I feel you have really changed. I used to think you were independent and strong. Lately you have become a dependent and you act like a child.
Therapist:	Explain to him why you perceive him as a child.
Marlene:	Your mother tells you what to do and when to do it. Ever since she moved in, she's taken over. She cooks your favorite meals, does your laundry, and tells our kids what to do. I hate being in the same house with this woman, and yet I feel guilty because she's your mother and she has nowhere else to go.
Therapist:	Wait a minute! Neither of you told me that Luke's mother moved into your family home. Did this happen about two years ago? Why is she living with you? How did this happen?
Luke:	Yes, as a matter of fact, she did move in two years ago. My father died suddenly, and my mother was all alone. I told her she could move in with us. She had nowhere else to go. She's my mother. I didn't think Marlene would have a problem with that. If it were her mother, I would have done the same.
Therapist:	Luke, did you thoroughly discuss this with Marlene before you invited your mother to live with you?
Luke:	Well, not exactly. We're both family oriented, and I knew she would be fine with my mother moving in.
Marlene:	Well, I was not fine. You never once consulted me. After she moved in, I told you I wasn't happy with the arrangement, but I was willing to experiment with it for a couple of months. Then I wanted both of us to reevaluate the situation. I know she's alone, but she's not an invalid. I'm so sick of hearing her tell me what you

need and do not need that I could scream. Remember when she screamed at Cindy for leaving her toys in the living room? I tried to explain that she was not finished playing, but she continued to yell at her. You didn't do a thing. You just sat there like a wimp. After the two months were up, I said it's not working. Yet, you still did nothing to resolve it. I love your mom, but her living under the same roof is ruining our relationship. I have asked you a million times to talk to her about her intrusiveness, but you don't seem to be man enough to stand up to your own mother.

Therapist: It looks like you both got to the root of your sexual problem pretty quickly. Remember when you told me that power existed in your relationship? That is certainly not the case. Marlene, you perceive Luke as being a powerless child. Yet, if you were powerful, you would have been able to empower him. And Luke, you said that you considered yourself to be powerful, yet you couldn't empower Marlene. And together, you lacked the power to discuss this matter with Luke's mother. From where I am sitting, your relationship lacks power. Luke, you are the one who created this mess; what do you think you need to do to regain your power and empower Marlene?

Luke: I can start by not staying in the position of a helpless child and have a talk with my mother about our living situation. Marlene is right, I am afraid of hurting my mom's feelings at the expense of my family's feelings. But to tell you the truth, I also hate our living situation. There is just not enough time for us.

After much discussion, Luke and Marlene decided to discuss the situation with Luke's mother and request that she move out. They came up with a plan to financially support her by buying her a condo close by. At our next session, I asked how it went.

Luke: We both sat down, and I told my mother it was time to arrange a different living situation. I was totally honest with her and said that although we loved her, we needed our own family space. I told her that we would take care of her financially. She shocked me when she agreed that the plan was a great idea. She confessed that she also wanted her space but was afraid of hurting our feelings. What a relief. She's moving out in six weeks, and we're all thrilled!

Marlene: *(laughing)* Why don't you tell the doctor what else happened?

Luke: *(also laughing)* Right after I told my mother that she had to move, Marlene said she wanted to speak with me privately. At first I didn't know what she wanted, until she escorted me into our bedroom and, well, you know.

Therapist: No Luke, I don't.

Luke: We made love and it was great! We've made love three times this week.

Therapist: Marlene, why do you think that after two years of being sexually turned off, your libido went from a 0 to a 10?

Marlene: Actually, I'm not sure. All I know is that, when I listened to Luke talking to his mother, he was loving but firm. He seemed so impressive, you know, not like a little boy. I got so turned on by his calm but strong manner that I could hardly stand it. It's like I've got my old Luke back. I just don't want him to get too used to this three-times-a-week deal!

Although sexual desire was restored, they had plenty of work ahead of them to maintain power and power reciprocity in order to keep their relationship on track.

Let's end this chapter by quickly taking a look at what was missing in their relationship when they initially entered therapy.

Individual Power

Did Luke possess individual power? Perhaps he was a powerful attorney, but as a son, he felt helpless. He never attempted to confront and voice his opinions to his mother, even when he saw that she was interfering with his marriage. As a result, Marlene viewed him as a mommy's boy and a wimp.

As for Marlene, she acted powerfully when she originally told Luke that she did not like this living situation, but he chose to ignore her. As a result, she stopped voicing her opinion, viewed Luke as weak, and became quietly angry and resentful. This rendered her powerless in her own mind, so it did not matter that Luke still perceived her as powerful. She saw herself as weak, and she saw her husband as weak.

Power Reciprocity

Did Luke empower Marlene? Not at all. Instead, he chose to ignore her initial requests. Did Marlene empower Luke? She made an initial try by asking him to do something about their living situation, but she quickly gave up and withdrew into herself. If neither had the ability to empower the other, there could be zero power reciprocity.

Sexual Desire

Without individual power and power reciprocity, their relationship inevitably suffered from a lack of sexual desire. How could Marlene feel desire for someone that she saw as a mommy's boy? However, once Luke reclaimed his individual power by speaking to his mother, which enabled Marlene to regain her own sense of power in her home, power reciprocity was restored. When power reciprocity was restored, Marlene's desire for Luke soared. After two years of not having sex, they had sex three times that week. That is because now Marlene not only viewed Luke as powerful and sexy, she saw herself as powerful as well, capable of persuading and influencing her husband to create a positive effect—the restoration of balance in their home.

Communication Skills

When they first came to see me, their communication skills were dismal. Both ignored each other, did plenty of mind reading, made little eye contact, and certainly did not actively listen or try to connect with each other emotionally. Neither shared their authentic feelings. As mentioned earlier, power reciprocity requires effective communication skills and connected conversations.

It's been five years since I saw this couple in therapy. They stay in touch and tell me that their sex life has been great ever since Luke stood up to his mother. You see, it doesn't matter how powerful you may be in the eyes of the rest of the world, it's how powerful you become in the eyes of your partner—and yourself—that counts in creating sexual desire.

Marlene and Luke are no different than most couples I have treated for a sexual desire disorder. While their loss of power may have originated in any number of life situations, they all have one thing in common; once they pinpoint what caused that loss of power and restore both individual power and power reciprocity to their relationship, sexual desire soars. And when desire is high, sex is fantastic!

At last, the part you have been eagerly anticipating. That's right, it's time to turn the knowledge that you've acquired so far into action.

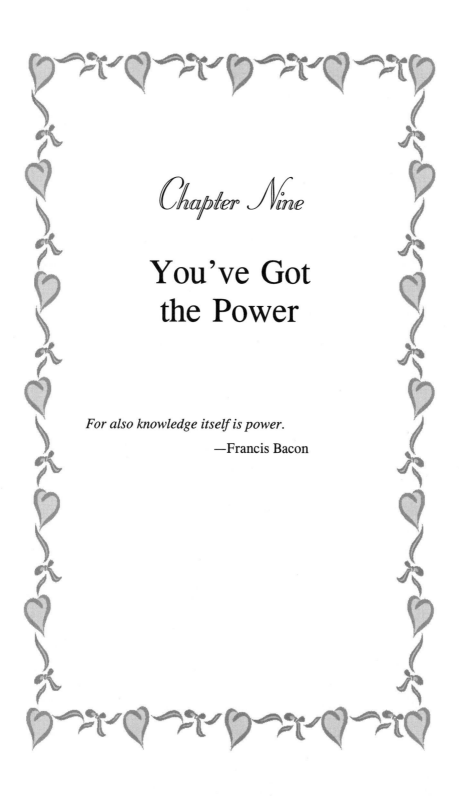

Chapter Nine

You've Got
the Power

For also knowledge itself is power.

—Francis Bacon

This exciting and fast-moving chapter marks the beginning of the action phase of therapeutic process.

Hang on to your hats; we'll move quickly. Each characteristic needed to develop the aphrodisiac of individual power will now be thoroughly examined and implemented. Developing or enhancing these characteristics will require a detailed conversation between you and your partner. As you are about to discover, this chapter contains a series of fun and stimulating exercises.

Let's briefly go over the definition of individual power. Individual power is being influential, impressive, persuasive, and having the capacity of producing a positive effect. Now, let's take a brief look at the characteristics needed to develop individual power. They are: integrity, humor, empathy, assertiveness, emotional awareness, autonomy, decisiveness, financial balance, and self-observation.

Before you and your partner engage in these exercises, I'd like you to take a good look around you; what do you see? It's an imperfect planet, where everybody in it has flaws. Society is flawed, you and I are flawed, and every relationship on this planet has flaws. With this in mind, I would like you to relax and not attempt to strive for perfection. People who believe in the existence of perfection become frustrated and exhausted by their attempt to achieve something that's impossible. Do not put that kind of pressure on yourself; be bold in your commitment for change but realistic in your immediate expectations.

A level of sexual desire, for example, can never be exactly what you and your partner would ideally like it to be. If I had my druthers, I would like my desire level to be high and ready to act on anytime I wished. That, however, is an impossible dream. Even if there were no obstacles interfering with sex motivation, which is impossible to begin with, there are too many other unknown variables that keep us from being a perfect 10 all the time. The exciting news is that you and your partner will be able to get back your sex life and maintain the desire level you once enjoyed before it took a nosedive. Actually, some couples have reported that they now have a higher sex drive than experienced in the past because they now have a clearer understanding of what is needed to increase desire. It's not perfection, but it is success!

Remember the euphoric lust phase? Most likely, both you and your partner fueled those flames of sexual desire by an unconscious use of power. You exuded individual power, and you exchanged that power without being aware of exactly what you were doing. That's how you managed to persuade one another to share the rest of your lives together. You have to admit that it was a monumental decision. You were able to produce a great effect on one another because you possessed and used the characteristics of power. As time progressed, your power in the relationship lacked the intensity it had in the beginning. You did not lose your individual power; it only became dormant. Don't worry, it happens to most of us. It's time to reawaken these characteristics of power. Once you develop your individual power, you will learn how to exchange it (chapter 10) and re-ignite the flame of desire. That's right, you'll be in the mood again.

Ground Rules for Exercises

Below I have listed the characteristics of individual power followed by a self-rating questionnaire. If you are currently applying one or more of these attributes of individual power, that's great. If, say, you are lacking one characteristic or feel you need to enhance it, face your partner and complete the following steps:

- *State the importance of this characteristic and what it means to your relationship.*

- *Describe a specific instance in your life where this characteristic was lacking, and what you lost because if it.*

- *Indicate to your partner how willing you are to add or enhance this characteristic in your relationship.* Be open and willing to share, but avoid any self-pity, guilt, or shame. Talk with a strong voice, sit erect, face your spouse, and maintain eye contact.

- *Ask your partner to repeat what you said.* If he or she misses something important, conclude that *you* did not make your message clear enough, rather than blame your partner for not listening carefully enough. Reexpress your message and have him or her repeat it.

Lastly, you and your partner must explicitly agree to the following:

- *Take turns.*

- *Do not interrupt each other.*

- *Don't judge or criticize.*

- *Don't withdraw or give up.*

- *Listen carefully to what the other has to say.*

Okay, let's get going and develop the characteristics of individual power.

Keeping Your Promise

Integrity is the internal characteristic of being trustworthy and honest. You are probably thinking, "Of course, both my partner and I are honest and trustworthy. Why would I remain in a relationship with someone I could not trust or believe?" You are right; however, did you know that if you say you are going to do something and you don't, you have just stepped out of integrity? I'll give you an example. When my husband and I did this exercise, he remembered the following incident and considered it an important turning point in our relationship. One evening, when we were dating, he said he would call me at 7:30. Instead, he called at 8:00, which he scarcely gave a second thought. Thinking I would be glad to hear from him, he was surprised to hear coldness in my voice, particularly when he didn't even bother with an explanation. While doing this exercise, he recalled that I told him I had postponed doing my laundry so I could be by the phone to take his call. I felt disrespected, angry, and disappointed. I explained that his lack of integrity made me feel unimportant and undervalued. He admitted that he never considered lateness as an integrity issue and apologized for the late phone call.

No matter how insignificant a particular situation may appear, if you do not follow through on a promise, you are out of integrity. What does integrity have to do with sexual desire? The next example illustrates how quickly sex centers can shut down.

Mary and Tim were preparing to celebrate their seventh wedding anniversary. Tim secretly planned a romantic evening that included dinner, dancing, and an overnight stay in one of the most exclusive hotels in the area. Although Mary knew of the plan, the details were a surprise. He told her to be ready by 7:00 P.M. Mary's anticipation grew as the day progressed. She was feeling good about herself and the situation at hand. As you know by now, feeling good stimulates the sex centers.

Around 6:00 P.M. Tim was faced with an office emergency that normally would have taken a few minutes but took over an hour to resolve. He got caught up in this crisis and forgot to alert Mary.

Mary, who was dressed and ready to go, had no idea Tim would be late. As the scheduled time approached, her excitement grew. Then ten minutes passed, followed by another twenty. You could hear the ticking of the clock. "Where is he? Maybe he was caught in traffic or had an accident." In a panic, she phoned his office. Although relieved that he was safe, she was furious that he hadn't alerted her of his lateness.

"Don't worry honey, I phoned the restaurant and rescheduled our reservation," he said.

Mary's response was, "Well, call them back. I'm not going any- where." She took off her dress, climbed into bed, and ordered a pizza. Even the flowers he brought home didn't change her disappointment. What started out to be an exquisitely romantic evening turned into one of anger and sadness. As you can see by this illustration, if you do not possess integrity, your power slips away. No power, no sexual desire. No sexual desire, no sex.

Integrity demands honesty and trust. Always state what you mean and mean what you say; that's power. Of course, there will be times when you will be out of integrity. It happens to all of us. During one of my phone contacts to my husband, I told him I was feeling amorous. He was filled with anticipation on his drive home. By the time he arrived, however, I lost my desire to make love. Between the time I hung up with my husband and his arrival home, I received upsetting news, caus- ing my sex centers to slam shut. Was I out of integrity? The answer is yes. I apologized and said we could make love the following morning. He had two choices; he could seduce me or wait until morning. We waited until morning.

On another occasion, I promised myself that I would quit smoking. I cheated and smoked an occasional cigarette. Was I out of integrity? Yes, I was. I broke my promise to myself. My point is, do not expect perfection regarding integrity. All you can expect from yourself is the awareness that when you slip out of it, you quickly apologize to yourself or your partner and return to integrity. Let's take a look at your own amount of integrity.

Exercise: Self-Integrity

- *I consider myself trustworthy.*

You: Yes   No   Your Partner: Yes   No

- *I view myself as a person of my word.*

  You: Yes   No   Your Partner: Yes No

- *My partner counts on me to follow through on a promise.*

  You: Yes   No   Your Partner: Yes No

- *I'm honest during our interactions.*

  You: Yes   No   Your Partner: Yes No

- *If I do not follow through on a promise, I take responsibility for this lapse in integrity and quickly apologize.*

  You: Yes   No   Your Partner: Yes No

Humor

Humor is an important component of power. I'm not talking about being a comedian. Being a comic is a gift very few people possess. Having a sense of humor, however, means that you have the ability to laugh at yourself and not take life so seriously. Usually people who are unable to laugh at themselves are defending against their flaws. To laugh at one's self is an admission of these flaws. The sooner you can admit to yourself that you are not perfect, the sooner you can have a good laugh at yourself. Years ago while giving a lecture, I mistakenly thought the lectern was glued to the desk that I was standing behind. I carefully placed my notes on the lectern and began my talk. I was moving right along but felt tired of standing so I leaned against it to get support. Then it happened. I leaned, it flew, leaving me sprawled across the desk with all my notes scattered all over the floor. The room became astoundingly silent. As I looked up, I saw a sea of faces straining against repressed laughter. At that moment, I began laughing and said; "Come on, let your laughter out; I'd be roaring on the floor if I were you." With this permission from me, the audience burst out laughing and at that instant, they all gave me a standing ovation. Did I feel powerful? Sure I did. I'm not perfect, and besides it was pretty funny.

Many individuals take themselves a bit too seriously while making love. Somehow, they think that they have to be perfect in bed. What a mistake this is. Sex therapists call this "performance anxiety." If you are concentrating on being perfect, you are taking yourself away from the sensual and loving experience. While lovemaking, one should never self-scrutinize. Instead, concentrate on those wonderful feelings your body is experiencing. Stay completely immersed in those sensual moments. Plus, sex is supposed to be fun.

When you notice your partner taking life a bit too seriously, help him or her get in touch with the humor of the situation. It helps to lift any type of humiliation experienced when bumping into an imperfection.

Exercise: Finding Humor Within

- *I have the ability to laugh at my imperfections.*

  You: Yes   No   Your Partner: Yes No

- *When I make a mistake I can quickly blow it off.*

  You: Yes   No   Your Partner: Yes No

- *While making love with my partner I often laugh at our blunders.*

  You: Yes   No   Your Partner: Yes No

- *My partner and I take enough time to play and have fun.*

  You: Yes   No   Your Partner: Yes No

- *When I notice that my partner is experiencing humiliation, I quickly do what I can to eliminate his or her shame.*

  You: Yes   No   Your Partner: Yes No

Empathy

Empathy is the ability to temporarily climb into your partner's mind and understand how he or she thinks and feels about certain situations. Being empathic involves work and concentration. The rewards, however, are plentiful. Why is empathy so important to sexual desire? If you understand your partner's point of view, you can be more influential, persuasive, and convincing while conveying your own point of view. It's a quid pro quo; if you take the time to understand your partner, your partner in turn will take the time to understand you. When you feel understood, your sex centers are open.

Most powerful people understand the importance of empathy. They make it a point to understand the people with whom they are interacting before they verbalize their point. Their motto is: Know who you are dealing with.

The reward is that you are meeting a basic human need; that is, to feel understood by another person. You have to admit, when you understand your partner, and he or she understands you, you will both immediately feel connected to each other. Sexual desire is sparked by feelings of connection to one another.

Exercise: Nurturing Empathy

- *I accept differences in my partner.*

    You: Yes   No   Your Partner: Yes No

- *Most of the time I feel understood by my partner.*

    You: Yes   No   Your Partner: Yes No

- *I am comfortable sharing my emotions with my partner.*

    You: Yes   No   Your Partner: Yes No

- *When my partner is upset, he or she can share that feeling with me.*

    You: Yes   No   Your Partner: Yes No

- *I take the time required to understand what my partner is feeling.*

    You: Yes   No   Your Partner: Yes No

Respect

Respect is honoring yourself and your partner. Respect means that you each treat one another with consideration and dignity. This does not mean that you have to agree with one another on all issues. That would be boring. You do, however, have to accept one another, flaws and all. We are all wired differently. You, for example, may approach life situations on an emotional level, while your partner prefers a factual level. Either way is fine, as long as you respect these differences. During the euphoric lust phase, you each valued and accepted one another's differences. I suggest you recapture that acceptance. If you try to change your partner, you are not honoring who he or she is currently.

I am certain that you have never observed a powerful person attempt to demean another. They may challenge and disagree with another's point of view, but they never diminish another during an interaction. If they do, they lose power. Belittling your partner will automatically decrease sexual desire. You will feel badly about yourself that you stooped so low, and your partner will feel humiliation. Disparaging behavior is powerless behavior. Join the ranks of powerful people by developing respect.

Self-respect is equally important to power. Love who you are and honor yourself. If you respect yourself, others will respect you as well. Have you ever seen powerful individuals demean themselves? They may apologize for mistakes made or laugh at their flaws, but they never make disparaging remarks against themselves.

Exercise: Cultivating Acceptance

- *I honor myself, flaws and all.*

  You: Yes No   Your Partner: Yes No

- *I honor my partner, flaws and all.*

  You: Yes No   Your Partner: Yes No

- *I treat my partner with the same respect that I would treat any other important person in my life.*

  You: Yes No   Your Partner: Yes No

- *My partner values my opinions.*

  You: Yes No   Your Partner: Yes No

- *When I challenge my partner's point of view, I never demean.*

  You: Yes   No   Your Partner: Yes No

Assertiveness

Assertiveness means that you actively take the bull by the horns. Being assertive means that you can boldly state what you want and achieve your goals with tenacity. A nonassertive person either avoids confrontation or is too nice. Assertiveness is commonly confused with aggressiveness. The difference is that aggressive individuals achieve their goals through disrespectful bullying. Assertive individuals achieve their goals with respect, dignity, and tenacity.

A nonassertive partner can be a sexual turnoff. It's the antithesis of power. Most individuals that I have interviewed stated that a passive man or woman screams powerlessness. I do not know many people who would view a submissive partner as sexy.

Exercise: Developing Initiative

- *I am comfortable with confrontation.*

  You: Yes   No   Your Partner: Yes No

- *I often turn down requests that I do not feel like granting.*

  You: Yes   No   Your Partner: Yes No

- *I usually feel good about myself after a heated argument.*

  You: Yes   No   Your Partner: Yes No

- *When I need a favor, I am comfortable requesting it.*

  You: Yes   No   Your Partner: Yes No

- *Most people would describe me as being assertive.*

  You: Yes   No   Your Partner: Yes No

Emotional Awareness

Being attuned to your emotions means that you are in touch with your feelings, thoughts, and desires; and you have the ability to openly discuss them with one another.

Women usually have an easier time expressing feelings than men do. This is due in part to both socialization and biology. Men, however, do have the capacity to discuss their emotions if their partner provides them with a supportive atmosphere. A powerful woman can empower a man in becoming emotionally aware. Once a man has experienced emotional awareness, he will be better equipped to empower his partner as well. Also, women should be honored that their man is willing to express a side of him that no one else ordinarily sees.

Keep in mind that unpleasant feelings will not go away magically. They need to be shared with your partner. Discussing negative feelings will alert you that action must be taken to change these feelings. If action is not taken, your desire will remain low until a more positive feeling reemerges. By the same token, getting in touch with positive feelings and expressing them will stimulate the sex centers, which keeps your sexual desire high.

Have you ever been around someone who cannot get in touch with his or her feelings? There is nothing more frustrating than trying to have a conversation with someone who is this powerless. The next example will illustrate this fact.

Tina and Thomas requested therapy because Tina had lost all desire for sex around eleven months ago. Thomas admitted that he was not as sexually attracted to her as in the beginning of their relationship. Thomas felt the reason for this was because Tina had become totally unresponsive to his sexual requests. They stated that they loved each other and would do anything to save their marriage. Thomas, however, stated that he felt that sex was part of a loving relationship, and without the intimacy of sex, he would be forced to request a divorce. I began the session by asking them to tell each other what they thought changed their sexual relationship.

Thomas: Why do you not want to have sex anymore?

Tina: I really don't know. All I know is that I'm no longer interested in sex.

Thomas: Do you feel that there are problems in our relationship that I'm unaware of?

| *Tina:* | I don't know. I wish I knew what the problems were so we could resolve them. |

| *Thomas:* | Tell me what you're feeling right now. |

| *Tina:* | I have no idea. I feel numb and shut down. |

Thomas continued to ask question after question, and she continued to respond with, "I don't know." He then exploded into a rage.

| *Thomas:* | If you don't have any ideas or opinions on what's going on, and you don't know what you are feeling or thinking, how can we work on our relationship? We might as well end it right now. |

Although I empathized with Thomas's frustration regarding Tina's lack of power, I have to point out that Thomas lacked individual power as well. If he possessed power, he would have been able to empower Tina by giving her more time to respond to his questions. He could have offered *his* perception of their current situation. In doing so, she might have been able to either agree or disagree with his assessment. Instead, he fired one question after the other in a rather accusatory and angry manner. This only served to reinforce Tina's powerlessness. The angrier he became, the more shut down she became, and the more she shut down, the more frustrated he became. Both were equally responsible for their unhappy situation. If either one could have tapped into their power, this cycle would have been broken.

Tina needed to get in touch with her feelings before she could voice them, which is not always an easy task. It takes courage to feel unpleasant emotions. Most of us would rather numb these feelings than to experience the pain they cause. Painful feelings, however, have valuable life lessons hidden inside. If Tina's feelings were painful, she needed to confront them head on. If she doesn't confront these feelings, how on earth can they resolve their issues? Thomas, on the other hand, needed to drop his defensiveness and voice what he was feeling and thinking about their present situation. All it takes is for one member of the relationship to tap into individual power and power reciprocity. This will clear the path needed for a connected conversation.

As you can see by this illustration, getting in touch with your emotions is important in a powerful relationship.

Exercise: Sharing Your Feelings

- *When I'm happy and excited, I share these feelings with my partner.*

  You: Yes   No   Your Partner: Yes No

- *If I feel anger, disappointment, or resentment, I tell my partner why I'm experiencing these feelings.*

  You: Yes   No   Your Partner: Yes No

- *During a painful event, like the death of a loved one, my partner and I can cry together.*

  You: Yes   No   Your Partner: Yes No

- *My partner and I often laugh together.*

  You: Yes   No   Your Partner: Yes No

- *I feel totally comfortable sharing most of my feelings with my partner.*

  You: Yes   No   Your Partner: Yes No

Autonomy

I have asked hundreds of men and women to define the most attractive trait found within a powerful person. The answer was always the same, "The most attractive trait is someone who knows who they are and is responsible for their own lives. They do not seem to depend on anyone else to fulfill their needs. They are able to make their own decisions and do not appear to need the acceptance or approval of others. Independent individuals do not depend on anyone to make them feel whole or to care for them."

There is a distinction, however, between needing something from your partner versus wanting something from him or her. For example, I am perfectly capable of making restaurant reservations, choosing that perfect hotel, and purchasing theater tickets. I do not *need* my husband to do those things. I am, however, one of those women who *wants* my husband to take charge once in a while. In other words, I empower him to do those things because of a request I made during one of our connected conversations. He said he would be happy to take charge as long as I did not complain about any of his choices. I happily agreed.

Independent people are powerful. Powerful people are sexy.

Exercise: Fostering Self-Reliance

- *I consider myself an independent person.*

  You: Yes   No   Your Partner: Yes   No

- *I make most personal decisions without my partner's permission.*

  You: Yes   No   Your Partner: Yes   No

- *I usually rely on my own good judgment.*

  You: Yes   No   Your Partner: Yes   No

- *If my partner left me, I would be sad but I could live life on my own.*

  You: Yes   No   Your Partner: Yes   No

- *I prefer spending free time with my partner.*

  You: Yes   No   Your Partner: Yes   No

Decisiveness

Decisiveness is having the power to think something through and then to make a decision. It's about making up your mind. It can be anything; you choose to go to one restaurant over another. You choose chocolate because that's what you like. You choose to be a ski instructor even though your parents wanted you to be a dentist. Powerful people are decisive. They know what they want and are determined to get it. Of course, in a relationship, decisiveness also means compromise. You can choose to have sex every night; however, if your partner chooses to have sex once a year, who is going to win? Both of you do if there is compromise.

If your partner asks, "Where would you like to go on vacation?" Give your answer. Don't go back and forth ad nauseam, "I don't care, where do you want to go?" Followed by, "Gee, I don't know. Where would you like to go?" Make a decision where to go and start packing. It is, however, important to make these decisions as a couple.

When you are indecisive, it can mean that you are afraid of making a mistake. We all make mistakes. Why should you be any different? If the decision you made about something is a wrong one, let it go and make a better one in the future. The important thing is that you become more decisive; it's powerful.

Exercise: The Power to Decide

- *I consider myself a decisive person.*

    You: Yes   No   Your Partner: Yes   No

- *My partner and I can make major decisions as a couple.*

    You: Yes   No   Your Partner: Yes   No

- *When we disagree on some issue requiring a decision, we can usually compromise successfully.*

    You: Yes   No   Your Partner: Yes   No

- *I enjoy the fact that my partner can make decisions whether they are right or wrong.*

    You: Yes   No   Your Partner: Yes   No

- *I'm comfortable with making decisions.*

    You: Yes   No   Your Partner: Yes   No

Although what I am addressing next is not a characteristic, it's not an obstacle either. It's in a gray area that is, however, important to address.

Financial Balance

I have observed couples where one member rides shotgun over the money. It's usually the partner who is earning more money. He or she usually feels that it's their privilege to say where and when the money is spent. In some cases, one partner actually decides to give the other a weekly or monthly allowance. I cannot think of anything more demeaning or invalidating to the partner who earns less or nothing at all. There are two extreme scenarios that I would like to address. Hopefully, you won't be able to identify with these situations. If you do, however, it's imperative that you change it immediately. Imbalance and power reciprocity are mutually exclusive.

The first scenario includes a subset of those couples who make the decision to have children. They agree that having a parent stay home with the child is beneficial to the child's welfare. Whoever that person may be, usually the woman, he or she gives up making a salary for the sake of rearing the children. Yet, if the stay-at-home parent were to be financially compensated for their work at home, they would be far from paupers—given the cost of child care and running a home. Rather than treat this person as contributing to the welfare of the family, a subset of such families either overtly or covertly treat the stay-at-home parent as unable to take on the financial responsibilities of an adult. The partner who earns the salary somehow feels justified in dictating where and when the money will be spent, and financial decisions are never shared.

This type of attitude and control causes an instant imbalance in the relationship. Reciprocity and disparity are totally opposing concepts. It is impossible for these concepts to exist simultaneously. If power reciprocity does not exist, sexual desire will be low or nonexistent. The so-called breadwinner may feel powerful because he or she is controlling the money, but at what expense? The partner not holding the purse strings will feel infantilized, resentful, and demeaned. What happens when we experience these feelings? Yes, sexual desire takes a nosedive.

The second scenario involves those couples where each earns a salary, but one earns more than the other does. Similar to those couples mentioned above, the partner earning more somehow feels entitled to call the financial shots.

The bottom line to both these scenarios is that there is an inappropriate imbalance of power. After all, a relationship is a partnership, and only by contributing both goods and services will a partnership survive. It simply doesn't matter who earns what. The point is that in a relationship, each partner needs to be treated as an adult who has an appropriate say in financial decision-making.

In most relationships, one person is often more knowledgeable about money, and it would be a mistake not to make use of the best person's expertise regarding investment, insurance, buying a home, saving for retirement, doing taxes, and making major or household purchases. However, every adult needs to learn about financial matters. After all, one day the spouse who handles all financial details may die, leaving the other financially and emotionally vulnerable. Just because your spouse is an expert in financial matters is no reason to avoid the adult responsibilities of finance.

What steps can be taken if your financial relationship is unequal? The one with less financial skill can learn from their partner, or better yet, take advantage of finance courses offered by cities or community colleges.

Sharing or having responsibility for part of the money is also important. One practical way you might consider is for each relationship to have three separate accounts. One would be a joint account out of which the household bills are paid. The other two would be individual accounts. Each person in the relationship can then use their equal share to spend or save in any way they wish. If you do not work out some arrangement of your money that involves both of your input, you are setting yourself up for resentment. No one enjoys asking a partner for money. If you are having money problems, seek out a financial counselor. Money conversations are usually volatile. A counselor can serve as a buffer and help prevent an explosive situation from happening.

Exercise: Maintaining Balance

- *I have meaningful decision-making responsibilities in all aspects of our financial dealings.*

  You: Yes   No   Your Partner: Yes   No

- *I feel that my partner and I have an equal financial partnership.*

  You: Yes   No   Your Partner: Yes   No

- *We live within our financial means.*

  You: Yes   No   Your Partner: Yes   No

- *When there are critical financial decisions to be made, we make them together.*

  You: Yes   No   Your Partner: Yes   No

- *I respect my partner's judgment regarding financial decisions.*

  You: Yes   No   Your Partner: Yes   No

Observing Your Own Behaviors

Powerful people are aware of how they present themselves to others. Here is how they develop this skill. Pretend that you have a helium balloon attached to your wrist and that balloon is *you* actually observing yourself. Every person has the capacity to do just that. Much of the time, however, this observation occurs on an unconscious level. An example of this is not picking one's nose in front of another. We may like to, but unconsciously we realize that this behavior would be rude, not to mention gross. What would happen if we started observing ourselves on a conscious level? The results would be awesome. Powerful people do just that. They are totally aware of how they are being perceived. They make an impression on another by producing a positive effect. They stand erect, speak clearly, are attentive listeners, smile freely, make penetrating eye contact, and stay focused on the issue at hand.

You and your partner exhibited these very same behaviors during the euphoric lust phase, remember? If you are not using these behaviors currently, pull them out and use them once again. It's a turn-on to be in the presence of someone who uses these behaviors.

Exercise: Respectful Behaviors

- *My partner would describe me as having good listening skills.*

  You: Yes   No   Your Partner: Yes   No

- *I'm usually attentive during a conversation with my partner.*

  You: Yes   No   Your Partner: Yes No

- *I'm usually interested in what my partner is saying to me.*

  You: Yes   No   Your Partner: Yes No

- *My partner would describe me as being friendly.*

  You: Yes   No   Your Partner: Yes No

- *I feel listened to by my partner.*

  You: Yes   No   Your Partner: Yes No

Congratulations, you are now aware of your individual power and you know how to tap into it. One last reminder: do not expect perfection. You cannot feel powerful every minute of every day. The important thing is to be aware that power exists within you to tap into anytime you wish. The more powerful you become, the more sexual desire you will have. Now, give yourself a big pat on the back and hug your partner. You both did a lot of work.

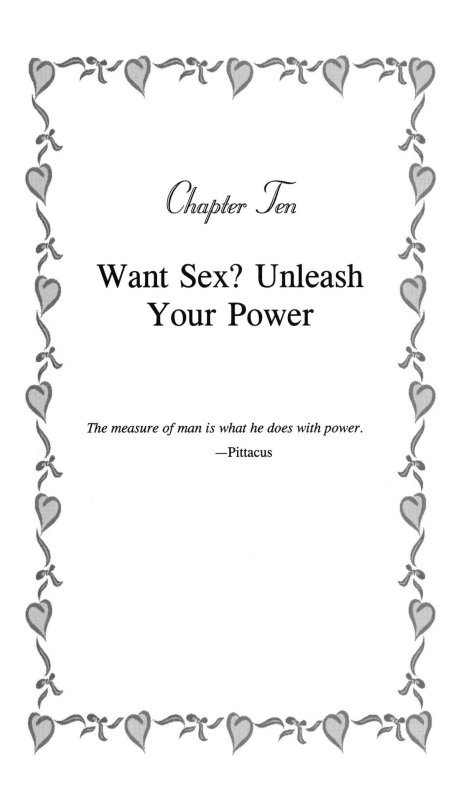

Chapter Ten

Want Sex? Unleash Your Power

The measure of man is what he does with power.

—Pittacus

Now that you are exquisitely aware of possessing individual power, you have to learn what is needed to exchange it. Once you learn the art of power reciprocity, your sex centers will spring to life.

The total concept of reciprocity is that you give to get. Whatever you give your partner, it will be returned to you. Whatever your partner gives you, you will return in kind. If your partner ignores you, you will most likely ignore your partner, and vice versa. If your partner is an enthusiastic lover, you will return the enthusiasm. If you, however, show little enthusiasm for making love, I am sure your partner will try to rush through lovemaking to put you out of your misery. Are you beginning to get the picture? You will get back exactly what you give, and your partner will get back exactly what he or she gives.

Power reciprocity is all about intention, enticement, persuasiveness, and seduction. On a nonsexual level, you do this every day. You want your kids to maintain good health so you seduce them into eating their peas; they eat their peas, and you in turn get to feel like a successful parent. You persuade your boss into thinking you are the best thing that ever happened to their company before you ask for a raise. The company offers you the raise and it gets a happy employee. During your courting phase, you enticed your partner into feeling that you, and only you, would enhance his or her life, and your partner did the same. You gave love, and it was returned. When it was returned, you returned it back and so on. That's power reciprocity. During each one of these transactions, you both had individual power that you were exchanging with one another.

Almost every single person I have ever treated for a sexual desire disorder temporarily lacks power and has a powerless partner. The bottom line is, for most people, a powerless individual is a sexual turn-off—plain and simple.

The irony is that every single person I have treated for a sexual desire disorder is partnered with a powerful person in every other way. They are able to successfully drive trucks, raise children, teach students, treat patients, win law cases, unclog drains, build houses, own businesses, just to name a few. Why do these powerful individuals turn into wimps when it comes to interacting with their partners? They lack intention and present themselves as ineffectual when engaged in an intimate conversation. A lack of sexual desire feeds on powerless conversations. We will explore connected conversations in more detail in the following chapters.

Let's take a look at the following illustration of a couple engaged in a conversation without power reciprocity. Then we'll look at the same conversation with power reciprocity.

Marcy and Max have been married for seven years. For the past two years, Marcy has lost all sexual desire for Max. I asked Marcy to tell Max what he could be doing to contribute to Marcy's lack of desire. She immediately figured out the two primary obstacles interfering with her sex centers. These obstacles were that she did not feel listened to and felt sexually objectified.

Without Power Reciprocity

Marcy: Max, you do not listen to me when I tell you what turns me off. You continue to make me feel like a sex object, even when I tell you to stop. So, I just stopped telling you, because it doesn't seem to matter.

Max: You never told me that I do things that turn you off. What are you talking about?

Marcy: This is embarrassing, but I'll tell you again. Every night, when I am rinsing off the dishes, you come up behind me and grab my breasts. I hate that. I told you a million times to stop, but you don't listen to me. I stopped telling you months ago because it doesn't do any good. Now I just grit my teeth until you eventually stop.

Max: My touching you makes you grit your teeth? That's just great. I think you are sexy and want to touch your breasts, and that makes you cringe? Would you like me to stop touching you? If that's what you want, I'll keep my hands to myself and never touch you again!

Marcy: That's not what I said. You just don't understand what I'm trying to say. You simply don't listen to me.

Max: It's hard to listen to you when you just told me that I make you cringe when I touch you.

Is this power reciprocity? Of course not. It is just a verbal exchange going nowhere. They will remain stuck in this powerless dance until one of them begins to empower the other. With this type of powerless exchange their sex centers will remain shut tight. This exchange lacked intention, purpose, and engagement. They were each defensive, angry, and whiney. Did Marcy get Max to take her request seriously? Did Max listen to or understand her request? Now, let's look at the same message delivered with power reciprocity.

With Power Reciprocity

Marcy: Max, we need to sit down and talk about something important that's been bothering me for months.

Max: Okay, what is it? You look serious?

Marcy: This is embarrassing for me to discuss, and I'm afraid that what I have to say will hurt your feelings. But it needs to be said, because I feel that this is what is causing me to lose my sexual desire. Every night when I am rinsing off the dishes, you come up behind me and grab my breasts. I hate that. I'm not sure why, but I do. I feel like you are treating me like a sex object, and it upsets me. I've asked you to stop, but you continue to do it anyway. When I get upset like that, I don't feel like making love. Do you understand what I am saying? Please understand that I love you, and I am not trying to embarrass you.

Max: Yes, you have asked me to stop grabbing you from behind. I thought you were kidding around. I had no idea that it bothered you so much. I think that you are cute and sexy, and all I want to do is touch you and get close. I didn't mean to treat you like a sex object. You are certainly more than a pair of breasts to me. I can't say that I totally understand this. Do you want me to not touch your breasts?

Marcy: No, I love it when you touch me, when I am feeling close to you. But when you grab me from behind, there's no feeling of intimacy connected to it. Maybe if you kissed me on the neck or if we had some type of close communication, I would feel more of an intimate connection to you.

Max: I never saw it from your point of view. I am different; I can feel intimacy just touching you. But if you need a kiss on the neck or close conversation, I'd be happy to do that.

See the difference when power reciprocity is present? There was intention; Marcy asked Max to sit down so they could engage in a serious discussion. She was bringing power to the table. Marcy's voice was clear, and she shared her feelings by stating that she was embarrassed and did not want to hurt Max's feelings. In doing so, she began to empower Max. In other words, she was letting Max know that his feelings were important to her. Max understood her message of concern and knew that he did not have to defend himself against any type of anger or resentment. Hence, he was open to what she had to say. Marcy was persuasive when she offered a possible explanation for not wanting Max to grab her from behind. She was seductive when offering him the option of having a close conversation or a kiss on the neck before he sexually touched her. Max empowered Marcy by letting her know that he was trying to see her point of view and agreeing to instill intimacy prior to a sexual touch. They were both able to unleash their individual power and exchange it. Okay, it is your turn to unleash your power on one another.

Unleash Your Power and Turn On the Heat

The manner in which your partner sees and hears you is the most important component of power reciprocity. I simply can't stress this enough. I am not suggesting that you be ever vigilant regarding how you are perceived by your partner every minute of every day. What I am saying, however, is you must be conscious of how your partner is seeing and hearing you when you are engaged in connected conversations.

Ask yourself this question. Am I being enticing, persuasive, influential, seductive, and effectual while interacting with my partner?

Here are a few simple tips to help you when you are exchanging power.

Know Your Partner

The most powerful people in the world take the time to research the person with whom they will interact. They do this to insure that their transaction will be successful. So, why not apply this axiom to relationships? It stands to reason that the more you know about one another, the more powerful your transaction will be. Every single day we are in the process of change as we respond to and interact with our external environment and our internal mental states. Take the time to get to know your partner again; it's fun and exciting.

Using the above illustration, Marcy tapped into one of the components of individual power: empathy. She did this when she acknowledged the possibility that Max would feel embarrassment about doing something that turned her off. It may be that three years ago she would not have considered his behavior to be demeaning. Or, maybe three years ago Max would not have felt embarrassed that he grabbed her. And who knows, maybe next week Marcy will want Max to grab her from behind. The point is that we change every single day. Make sure you know your partner.

Create an Atmosphere of Intention

A lack of desire is a serious matter that requires an intimate and connected conversation. Any transaction regarding this issue has to have sensitivity, purpose, and design.

Intention means that you have some plan of action. Marcy had intention when she informed Max that they were about to engage in a conversation that was serious in nature. Max knew, by the look on her face, that they were about to discuss something meaningful. Because of this aura of intention, they were able to powerfully resolve the obstacle. Once they removed that obstacle, sexual desire was restored.

Before engaging in a serious conversation, you have to have a plan of action. How do you do this? Fast-forward yourself into the future. Think about the best possible outcome that can result from your upcoming discussion. Then ask yourself, "What did I say that mattered? How did I say it? What were the issues I addressed?" After you think this through, take action and have that conversation in the here and now. During that conversation, do not allow yourselves to be derailed regarding the issue at hand. Stay on the topic.

Be Aware of Your Body Language

Picture you and your partner engaged in this important conversation. Are you going to pay attention if he or she is curled up in a ball, looking defensive? Is your partner going to take this conversation seriously if your arms and legs are crossed and your head is hanging towards the floor? The answer to both questions is most likely no. This type of body language evokes sympathy, pity, or boredom. Human nature dictates that when someone looks or acts meek and unassertive, our response will be a sexual turnoff.

Sit straight, shoulders back, and uncross your arms and legs. Let your body express the powerful person that you know you are. Your message cannot be powerful unless you exhibit powerful body language.

The other side of the coin is exhibiting offensiveness. Leaning forward and making a fist with your hands manifest threatening body language. I can guarantee that neither of you will be receptive to any message while feeling at risk. If you do feel yourself getting offensive, lean back and relax your muscles before talking to your partner.

Observe Your Own Facial Expression

I was watching a daytime talk show that was discussing the topic of sexual dysfunction. A woman explained how she couldn't care less if she ever had sex with her husband again. As she made this declaration, the camera pointed to her husband. I considered him handsome and impeccably groomed. He did, however, look powerless. His eyes were cast downward, his mouth was turned down, and his posture stooped. He looked as if he could burst into tears any second. Of course, he was saddened by his wife's message that she no longer wanted to be sexual with him. I would have felt sadness as well. He stated that even his coworkers noticed that he was no longer his "cheerful self." He was facially showing the world his powerlessness.

He was then encouraged to enter a dialogue with his wife to try to begin to remedy their desire issue. During this dialogue, he continued to look ashamed. Maybe his coworkers were moved by his saddened facial expression, but his wife was not. I felt like he needed a nurturing hug. You can't be sexually turned on if a facial expression evokes a mothering response. Again, I am not suggesting that you can't facially express sadness when you are experiencing this feeling. Expressing the sadness you feel is absolutely appropriate, but another mood will need to take its place in order for you to look powerful in your partner's eyes. A powerful facial expression is part of power reciprocity. Maintain eye contact and be intentional about being powerful. It goes almost without saying, it is impossible to offer power to your partner when you do not possess it yourself.

The other side of the coin is facially exhibiting a look of anger, contempt, boredom, or disgust. When you roll your eyes or they are narrowed, I guarantee your partner will ignore your message. Sarcasm may be fun to see at the theater, but its aim is to belittle, a feeling incompatible with power. In an intimate and connected conversation with your partner, anger is counterproductive; it represents a loss of control rather than power. No person likes to feel intimidated; it's just not powerful.

Improve Your Voice Intonation

I'll get right to the point. A whiney voice is a major sexual turnoff. Plus, you simply cannot have a serious conversation with someone who sounds childlike. It is especially true with how women perceive men with whiney voices. Of course it is annoying when men hear women with wimpy voices as well.

I consider a clear and distinct voice as being paramount to power reciprocity. My private practice attracts some of the most influential and powerful professionals from all over the country. Yet, during their couple sessions, many of these powerful men whine when they explain to their partners how important sex is to their relationship. I watch the faces of these women as their partner whines away, and they exhibit disgust. I am pretty good at reading faces; after all, it is what I am paid to do. Yet, when I ask the woman what she was feeling when her partner was speaking, she generally clams up. I can understand this. After all, it is a difficult thing to have to tell your male partner that his voice sounds wimpy. When I get her alone in a session, however, the truth comes out. She states that his whiney voice reinforces her lack of sexual desire. So, I am telling all the men out there to observe their voice intonation.

Men are also turned off sexually by women with whiney voices, but not for the same reason. Men appear to conceptualize this as a little girl trying to manipulate a situation. Either way, a whiney voice is a turnoff. An easy way to help you hear yourself is to ask your partner to let you know when your voice appears whiney.

Become Persuasive

To persuade means to get your partner to do or believe something. You have to be convincing. It is totally up to you to get your partner to listen to you. Do not expect your partner to have mental telepathy. It is impossible to read someone else's mind; I don't care how long you've been together, your assumptions could be completely wrong. I can almost guarantee that assumptions can really lead to problems.

A case in point involves a couple named Linda and Lenny who had been married for twenty years. As Linda approached fifty, Lenny asked her if she would like him to throw her a birthday party to mark this special occasion. Linda told him that she'd rather let this birthday go unnoticed. Lenny listened to her request, and they spent a quiet day celebrating alone. Internally, she was disappointed that a surprise party was not held. She felt that Lenny should have known that she really wanted a birthday bash. Her disappointment led to anger. As a result, this couple did not have sex for eleven months. By the time they entered therapy, Linda didn't know why her libido was at an all-time low. When we finally got down to the obstacle causing her low desire and they each tapped into power, they were able to powerfully discuss it and her sexual desire returned.

Here is the crux of it: just because they were married for twenty years didn't mean mind reading was an option. Linda could have stated that it was embarrassing to request her own birthday party, but what the heck, let's have one anyway. That would have been direct and honest. On the other hand, did you perceive Lenny as being persuasive when he asked Linda if she wanted a party? I don't think so. He asked the question without any attempt to persuade Linda that it would be fun to celebrate her birthday. He could have empowered Linda into feeling excited about her big day. At the core, however, it was not his responsibility. It was Linda's responsibility to be clear and honest about her needs.

Processing Style Differences

For our purposes, to process means to think something through logically. Some individuals process quickly and some slowly. Do you think one way is better than the other? Some feel that if you process quickly, you are either a genius or careless. Some feel that if you process slowly, you are either brilliantly methodical or dense. Which way do you tend to lean? Regardless of your natural inclination, both ways are equally valid.

It is essential, however, that you know how you and your partner tend to process. If you process quickly and your partner processes more slowly, this difference in cadence can lead to annoyance and aggravation. This, of course, can cause problems in the relationship.

I remember treating a couple that actually argued because of the manner in which they each processed things. She accused him of being passive-aggressive because he took forever to respond to a question that required problem solving. He accused her of rudeness, because she interrupted him before he completed his response to solving a problem. He felt that she was sabotaging any type of problem solving because she arrived at solutions too quickly, and she thought that he was passive-aggressive, because he responded so slowly. The truth was that they both arrived at a similar resolution to problems at the same time. The quick processor will usually have to backtrack and the slower one has already methodically left no stone unturned.

Understanding Gender Differences

It is important to understand gender differences when interacting in a heterosexual relationship. We do not have to address the biological, hormonal, and intellectual differences between the sexes, because it's not relevant to power reciprocity.

There are a few areas where gender norms can affect your relationship. For example, we often think that males in our society are not permitted to express emotions. Actually, men are freely permitted to express anger, but not sadness or pain. Mainstream Western culture, however, has conditioned men to hide these feelings of vulnerability.

Somehow, our culture decided that it is more manly not to openly show emotion. This is not the case in other cultures. In my travels to other countries, I was struck by these cultural differences. There are cultures where men hug one another, cry openly when touched by something sensitive, and openly discuss feelings. Actually, there are cultures where men are openly affectionate and kiss each other on the mouth. Does that mean they lack power? No, of course not. We have all witnessed many powerful men openly express sadness and tears after a tragic event. My point is that both men and women have similar feelings. The difference is men and women may express them differently.

The overt expression of feelings, however, is not as important as being able to discuss these feelings.

For our focus, one of the important differences between the sexes is how they each experience sexual desire. I am not quite certain if it's nature or nurture that threw us this curve, but it can create severe problems within relationships.

Men do not need too much coaxing when it comes to being sexually turned on. All they seem to need is visual stimulation or a sexy thought to throw their sex centers into action. In addition, being sexual with their partner is a vehicle to feeling connected and intimate. If they have a willing partner and they are in good physical health, they usually can have sex anytime and anywhere. It is not being turned on that is their problem; it's being turned off that often decreases their desire. If their partner is critical, resentful, or demeaning (components of powerlessness), their sexual desire will become diminished. That makes perfect sense.

Although women are visually turned on as well, that's not usually the main thing that turns women on. Women seem to need intimate conversation and touching. It seems to take women more time to get in the mood. Engaging in sex is an *outcome* of the intimacy experienced in the kitchen, not in the bedroom. Once this piece of information is offered to couples, they seem to understand that on the whole, both sexes have more similarities than differences. Personally, I feel that it's a cop-out to focus on gender differences; it gives us permission to remain polarized.

Acknowledging Your Partner's Positive Attributes

Every day I observe couples engaging in powerless game playing. I recall telling a friend that I thought her husband was attractive. She said, "Yes, he is adorable, but don't ever tell him that, he'll get a big head." I asked her why she didn't let him know how handsome she thought he was. She said, "Well, he might think he can do better than me, and besides, he never tells me that I'm attractive." How on earth can your sex desire be turned on if you and your partner never offer positive feedback to the other? If you think your partner is smart, humorous, kind, attractive, generous, gentle, hardworking, sensitive, or any other trait you feel he or she possesses, state it verbally. Don't play games. If you and your partner have failed to acknowledge or compliment one another's attributes, I suggest that you be the one to break this powerless cycle. I promise, if you begin to acknowledge your partner's greatness, your efforts will be reciprocated.

Bravo! You are now aware of the concept of power reciprocity. I can see your sexual desire begin to increase as we speak. Now, take a break. You are almost there. I applaud your courage and all the work you and your partner have accomplished.

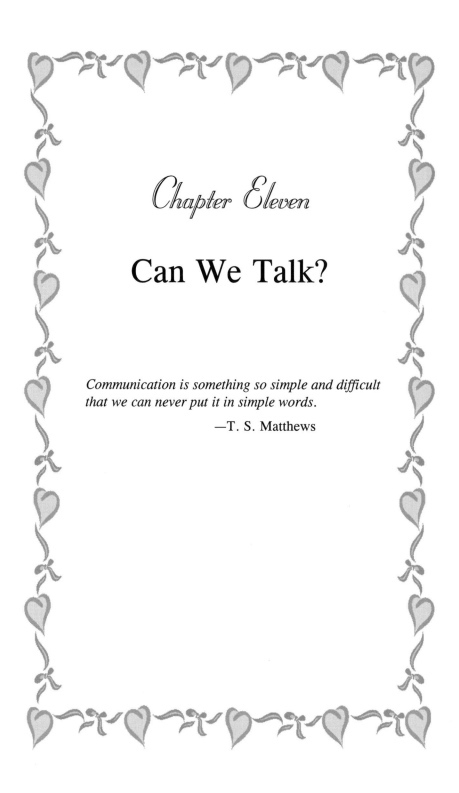

Chapter Eleven

Can We Talk?

Communication is something so simple and difficult
that we can never put it in simple words.

—T. S. Matthews

I'm certain that you and your partner talk, but do you really understand what the other is actually saying? Remember when you were young and played that telephone game? You and a bunch of friends sat in a circle. The first person began by whispering a message in the ear of the person to the right. The next person would whisper what they heard to the person to their right, and so on. By the time the initial message was received by the last person in the circle, the message was said out loud. The fun of this game was that the final message was unrecognizable from the original one.

Although this process caused uproarious laughter, it's no laughing matter when your partner misinterprets the meaning of your message, and vice versa. Actually, misunderstandings are one of the primary causes leading to low sexual desire.

Misunderstanding causes frustration and disappointment. Yet, nothing in the world is more difficult than trying to get your partner to understand you completely. Think about the complexities that the brain has to accomplish in order to translate a thought or feeling into language. You initially have a thought or feeling that you would like to express. You then have to translate this thought into words. Here's the hard part; once those words are spoken, you have to make sure that your partner actually understands the *meaning* of your words. It's totally your responsibility to make sure that your partner understands what you are trying to convey. A tip is to ask your partner, "Did you understand what I just said?" Or, "Did that make sense to you?" If you didn't quite understand your partner, ask, "Is this what you mean?" If you are like most couples, you are not doing this currently. That's okay; you are among the millions of people that didn't know you needed instruction as to how to talk. And I'm about to offer you just that!

Effective Communication

The following information describes the concrete skills of communication needed to be able to engage in a connected conversation. A connected conversation is the most powerful transaction that is absolutely required for sexual desire to be increased. You will soon discover, in the following chapter, exactly how to engage in this most intimate of all conversations. But first, you need to learn the basic skills of effective communication.

- **Sit Facing One Another.** It's best if you're seated at a table. Any place is fine, with the exception of the bedroom. The bedroom is a place reserved for lovemaking, not discussing issues. Why, you ask? You don't ever want any negativity or tension that conversations can produce to be paired with your lovemaking room. This room is sacred.

- **Maintain Eye Contact.** Penetrating eye contact is power.

- **Keep Your Voice Intonation Powerful.** Remember what you learned in the last chapter; neither of you will respond powerfully to a whiney or angry voice.

- **No Name-Calling.** A powerful person does not resort to debasing language.

- **Don't Mind Read.** Unless you possess psychic abilities, you cannot possibly know what the other is thinking; I don't care how long you've been together. Do your best to not assume anything; it is always problematic.

- **Use "I" Messages.** While discussing any issue, you must take total responsibility for your own thoughts, feelings, and opinions. To insure this, begin each statement with the pronoun "I" instead of "You." For example, "*You* make me angry when you want to have sex after an argument." This statement implies that your partner is responsible for your anger. Your partner certainly did not want to evoke an angry response. He or she wanted sex. The natural outcome of using "you" will be a defensive response from your partner. Instead, take responsibility for your own feelings, thoughts, and opinions. "*I'm* feeling angry that you want to have sex after an argument." Rather than evoking a defensive response, it will be more of an inquiry like, "Why are you angry? Will you explain why my wanting to make love makes you angry? I don't understand." After all, it's not your partner's requesting sex that made you angry. It was the fact that you did not feel an intimate connection that is necessary for making love.

Exercise: Listen Up

Now that you have the basics, let's get on with your basic interaction. Choose a sexual topic that you feel you would like to discuss for your interaction. Now, flip a coin to determine who will talk first. This keeps

it equal. Make sure that you time the interaction. Get a watch or an egg timer and place this in the middle of the table. Set the timer for three minutes.

You're probably thinking, "An egg timer, you have to be kidding?" Nope, I'm not. It's been my experience that one partner seems to monopolize a conversation. A three-minute limit will insure that you each have the same amount of time to make your point.

You have three minutes to deliver your message without any interruptions from your partner. Your partner will be forced to listen without any comment at all. Why is this so important? It's impossible to speak and listen at the same time. Most of us, while listening to a message, are also busy formulating a response. In doing so, we miss at least fifty percent of what was said. This technique will force you to be a better listener.

After your three minutes are up, ask your partner what you said. Your partner has to repeat what he thought he heard you say. If your partner gets it right, you can move on. If not, you have to repeat your message as many times as needed until it is finally understood.

Once your message is understood, it's your partner's turn to speak for the three minutes and you can't interrupt. You have to continue doing this until your discussion is over.

Here are two short examples illustrating ineffective and effective communication.

Ineffective Communication

Sally: I feel that you use sex as a way to resolve problems in this relationship. I can't be sexual if I don't feel intimate and connected to you.

Sam: (the listener offers his feedback) I don't feel that I use sex as a problem solver. I just want to be close to you because I love you.

As you can see, Sam responded to Sally's message rather than repeating back what Sally said.

Effective Communication

Sally: I feel that you use sex as a way to resolve problems in this relationship. I can't be sexual if I don't feel intimate and connected to you.

Sam: What I heard you say is that you feel I use sex as a way to resolve our problems. You don't feel that there is intimacy in this relationship. Is that what you said?

Sally: Yes, you heard me correctly.

This time Sam correctly repeated Sally's message rather than forming his own response.

Now it is Sam's turn as the speaker and Sally is the listener. You must continue in this highly mechanical manner until your conversation is completed. Once you get the hang of it, this technique will become second nature to you and you can lose the egg timer and the mechanical style.

Intensive listening is hard work. You have to practice creating an absolute blank slate mentally to truly receive your partner's message. The rewards of intense listening are many. Your partner will open up and share more information when you make an attempt to understand exactly what your partner is trying to say. And when you feel listened to, you will experience those same positive feelings as well.

Okay, now that you have the basic communication skills under your belts, let's take a look at how you put them together. Let's begin to develop conversational skills.

Conversational Skills

It is important to distinguish between a fight and an argument. I often hear couples proudly announce that they don't have arguments. My response to this is, "Really? That's too bad. I'll help you learn how to have them." Needless to say, they are confused by my response. Most couples believe that nice people don't argue. Or, they may be fearful that if they argue, they may hurt one another's feelings or experience anger. Their partner might think they are rude. Or, they feel that they are too timid to argue. Their partner might think they are either opinionated or an arrogant know-it-all. The list of excuses goes on and on. However, these excuses will stop this couple from being powerful.

Healthy Arguments

I personally don't know of any loving couple that doesn't argue from time to time. Arguing is healthy for a relationship. It allows you and your partner to know exactly where you each stand on an issue. As long as you are aware that you and your partner have a right to express feelings, values, opinions, beliefs, and grievances, and you each validate the other, it is a healthy argument. You don't have to agree with your partner's opinions, but you have to accept that your partner has the right to express them.

Most couples confuse an argument with a fight. Let's make a distinction between the two.

What Is a Fight?

It's the antithesis of an argument. During a fight, partners engage in the most disrespectful exchange in order to make the other wrong. Engaging in a fight is by far the most powerless conversation. Some partners will bully, badger, manipulate, control, name-call, yell, blame, and intimidate in an attempt to make their point. Usually, one person will feel defeated and leave the scene. A fight produces a winner or a loser. The person left standing has the misguided assumption that they won. The irony is, after the fight has ended, both individuals have lost, because the conflict was not resolved.

What Is an Argument?

An argument is a stimulating, passionate, exciting, and powerful process where you and your partner engage in an intimate and connected conversation with the sole intention of resolving conflict. The argument can be a difference of opinion or a grievance that needs to be resolved. Once you integrate the information throughout this chapter, you will find that you have all the skills needed to help you have successful arguments. Remember, there are no losers in an argument, and resolution is accomplished.

Let's explore the difference between a fight and an argument. I honestly wish I could tell you that the following illustration is rare. Actually, it's quite common. The good news is that fights can be turned into arguments with little effort. Fights are only manifestations of frustration and misunderstanding. When couples fight, it doesn't mean that they are bad or unloving individuals, it only means that they use bad and unloving techniques of communication. Once they learn effective techniques, they quickly switch to arguments.

Wendy and Hank exemplified this. They were great people who truly loved each other. However, their frustration reached a boiling point during their first session. Wendy was upset because Hank doesn't spend enough time talking to her. Hank was upset because Wendy was disinterested in sex. I'll illustrate, in parentheses, some of the negative techniques they each used.

Therapist: I'd like you to face each other. Flip a coin to decide who starts. Okay Wendy, tell Hank what you feel is causing problems in your relationship.

Wendy: *(Angry and screaming voice)* You don't care about me anymore. *(Mind reading. Hank never said that he didn't care about her.)* In the past you would talk to me for hours. Now all you want to do is sit and watch TV when you come home from work, then you want to go upstairs and have sex. You're boring and I'm sick of it. *(Name-calling)* If things don't change, and you don't start spending more time with me, I'm going to leave this relationship. *(Threatening and manipulative)*

Hank: *(Screaming and angry voice)* If that's what you want, I'll end this right now. I'm sick of your threats. If you want to leave, go ahead and leave. *(Threatening and manipulative)* You haven't loved me for months. *(Mind reading. She never said that.)* If you don't love me, there's nothing I can do about that." *(Zero power. He's defending himself by attacking her back.)*

Wendy: *(Whiney voice)* I didn't say that I didn't love you. I do love you, but you ignore me all the time. *(Zero power. She continues to attack. All she did was to change her voice from angry to whiney.)*

Hank: *(Angry voice)* I don't see how you can say you love me if you think I'm so damned boring, and you don't show me love. *(Zero power. His voice is intimidating.)*

I'm sure you get the point. Would you be persuaded to listen to either one of them? They used every powerless technique in the book. I, however, allowed them to continue this fight for a few more minutes. Although they were exchanging thoughts, feelings, and opinions, power was totally missing. When power is missing; it's a fight. Neither used their voice to be persuasive. How on earth did Wendy think that she would get her needs met by attacking Hank? And how did Hank think he could get her to feel loved when he was screaming? I finally intervened to turn their fight into an argument.

Now, let's take another look at Wendy and Hank in an illustration of an argument, not a fight. After three weeks of teaching them how to develop individual power, power reciprocity, and how to engage in a connected conversation, they were ready to begin to air their grievances in a powerful manner. The following is a short excerpt from their session. Wait until you see the transformation of this couple! They had the same problem to solve, but they each approached it with power.

Wendy: Do you remember when we used to talk for hours? I really enjoyed that and felt so close to you. I miss those talks because I love you. I realize that you enjoy watching TV, but I would like to have more of your time when you come home from work. I feel ignored. I sometimes don't feel like you love me anymore, and that scares me. I don't want our marriage to end. (*That was powerful.*)

Would you be persuaded to listen to that? Of course you would. The request was authentic, supportive, loving, and persuasive. It was powerful because the request was worthy of being listened to.

Hank: I do love you. I didn't realize that I've been ignoring you. I've been so busy at work and the kids need so much attention that watching TV relaxes me. But I see your point. Maybe I have been ignoring you. I don't want our marriage to end either. You have to understand my feelings also. I've felt ignored and rejected by you. For months you haven't wanted me near you sexually. That makes me scared. Having sex is a way to get close to you. (*That was powerful.*)

Arguments are great. How else can two separate individuals resolve conflict? We all have conflict in our relationships. If you don't, you're either denying it or avoiding it.

Okay, let's move on to the next conversational skill to develop.

Validate One Another's Perceptions

A perception is your own personal view of how you see and experience things. For example, after making love, your partner says,

"Wow, that was one of the best experiences I've ever had." You, however, may not have perceived this sexual experience as being all that great. Although you might not have perceived the experience as that great, you certainly don't have the right to invalidate your partner's perception of the experience. Yes, his or her experience was quite different from yours, but was it wrong? Of course not. There are no wrong perceptions.

For example, if you and your partner went to see a movie, and you loved the film but your partner hated it who is right? Yes, you are both right. You each have the right to your own perception.

I see plenty of couples trying to tell each other that their perceptions are wrong. Perceptions may be different, but not wrong. The key is that you don't have to agree with a perception; however, you do have to validate the fact that your partner has a right to his or her perceptions.

Powerfully State Your Feelings, Thoughts, and Opinions

As you already know, you have the right and the responsibility to state your personal feelings, thoughts, and opinions. Yet, you're faced with the arduous task of finding the words necessary to translate these emotions, thoughts, and opinions into language. For example, let's say that you absolutely hate liver; it disgusts you, and you wouldn't eat it for any amount of money. That's a strong emotion of hate and disgust, right? You and your partner go to a restaurant for a nice romantic dinner where liver is their specialty. Your partner turns to you and says, "Honey, are you going to try the specialty?" You think he's being humorous and reply, "Oh sure, I'd love to try the liver." He thinks you're being sincere. The waiter arrives and your partner orders, "We will both have the specialty." You say, "No, we won't! I'll have the lobster." Now, what do you think will happen next? Yes, a huge argument will ensue. You'll say something like, "I can't believe that we've been together for five years, and you don't know a thing about me; I hate liver with a passion." Your partner might respond, "How am I suppose to know you hate liver; the topic never came up. I took you at your word; you just said that you'd love to try the liver." You then respond, "I was being sarcastic; don't you recognize sarcasm?" He then responds in kind with, "I thought you were being sincere."

Now, the two of you are not talking about liver at all; you're accusing him of not knowing you at all, and he's confused about your verbal message being that you'd love to try the liver. The meaning was lost in the message. Will your evening be ruined? You bet it will. In addition, that romantic evening just went down the tubes and your sex centers slammed shut. What happened? The meaning of your message was misinterpreted. And your partner couldn't distinguish sarcasm from your true feelings. As mentioned, say what you mean and mean what you say.

Don't Allow Derailment

Let's assume that you are having a connected conversation about a particular grievance you may be harboring. As you begin to confront this grievance, your partner attempts to turn the tables on you, and begins to confront you with a similar grievance: "Oh yeah, you did the same thing to me last week." What do you do? Tell your partner that you are not addressing his or her complaint, but your own. Don't allow yourself to become sidetracked. Stay on task until your complaint is resolved. You can assure your partner that you will be happy to address his or her complaint after yours is resolved.

Remain in the Here and Now

During a connected conversation, not only should you stay on task, but you should remain in the present as well. It serves no purpose when you muddy the waters by bringing up unresolved incidents from the past. Trust this psychotherapeutic axiom. If an issue from the past went unresolved, believe me, it will come up again and again, until it finally seeks out resolution in the present. A grievance will not go away until it is resolved. It serves no purpose to discuss a missed opportunity from the past. Stay in the present.

Don't Be Afraid of Conflict

Keep in mind what I mentioned earlier: conversations are not always the warm and loving exchanges that we'd like them to be. They can be filled with disagreement. Disagreement doesn't mean that you don't love each other, it means that you possess the individual power to voice your disagreement. Embrace conflict; don't be afraid of it. The result from resolving any conflict is immensely rewarding. You will keep your relationship exciting, passionate, and authentic.

Recognize Your Partner's Conversational Style

Your partner may or may not converse in a style that is typical of his or her gender. The idea of gender-specific conversational style has never resonated with me personally. It is better to recognize the different styles and identify those components your partner and you tend to use.

Men are said to communicate in a pragmatic, intentional, and succinct manner. They like to get to the point quickly. They often look for problems to solve inside of most conversations. You'll often hear males make remarks like, "Will you please get to the point." Or, "Is this conversation going to last forever?" Or, "What's the bottom line?" Or, "I see the problem, why don't you try doing this."

Women are said to be loquacious, convoluted, detailed, and take forever in making their point. They enjoy conversing for the sole intention of sharing feelings, having fun, and because of the emotional connection it provides. Often their point gets lost in the verbosity of the interaction. Problem solving is not primary. That's not to say that women aren't problem solvers, because they are when the situation calls for it. You often hear women say, "How did you feel about that?" Or, "That must have hurt you." Or, "I had a similar feeling." Or, "What else happened?" Offering advice is not their primary intention.

Take these as gross characterizations of males and females. Your partner may follow these general patterns more or less, and his or her style may change depending on the setting. How can these different patterns interfere with you and your partner having a connected conversation? Women typically complain that men don't share enough and often withdraw from a conversation. Men typically complain that women belabor issues to the point of irritation. The solution is to use the best features of each style, as you will learn in the next chapter.

Lastly, I want to state that all individuals, including myself, have a limited attention span. After listening for so long, we seem to mentally go away. Therefore, both parties need to make their point as quickly and concisely as possible, before your partner's concentration level is depleted.

Bravo! You have both accomplished a great deal. You are amazingly close to regaining your sexual desire. It's time for a well-deserved break, because you'll need energy for this final and exciting phase. You are about to learn what a connected conversation entails and how to engage in one.

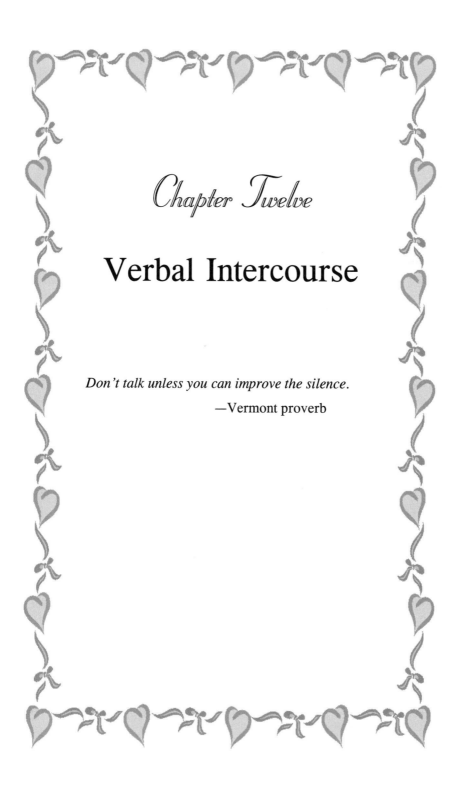

Chapter Twelve

Verbal Intercourse

Don't talk unless you can improve the silence.

—Vermont proverb

Verbal intercourse is any type of language exchange between two or more individuals. And I didn't make this up; it's in the dictionary. Verbal intercourse, as in sexual intercourse, can be filled with passion, intimacy, and love. Sometimes the experience can be fun and lighthearted. Or, it can be wildly passionate. Or, it can be warm and sensual. Of course, you determine the outcome by the amount of energy and time you're willing to invest.

How can you and your partner experience the close intimacy and passion that verbal intercourse can provide? It's simple: through engaging in connected conversations.

Just as we are not born with a sex manual, we are not given a manual that teaches us how to have connected conversations. That's why millions of couples are not enjoying verbal intercourse. In the previous chapter, we learned how to communicate effectively. Now we have to take those skills to a higher level, and that requires training.

In order to totally restore your sexual desire to the highest level possible, you must possesses individual power and exchange that power within a connected conversation. Remember, there will be little or no motivation for a physical connection if you don't have a connected conversation. Before we move on, we need to distinguish a connected conversation from the two more common types of conversations, the casual and informational.

The Casual Conversation

This type of conversation is filled with data regarding anything that doesn't directly relate to your relationship. It has no particular purpose, other than the sheer enjoyment of speaking to each other. It's fun to engage in a casual conversation, because you don't have to listen intently to every word your partner is saying. Your words flow quickly and easily. They go something like this, "Hi, honey, guess what? I finally got that promotion today. We can now afford that vacation we wanted. Let's celebrate and go out to dinner tonight. So, tell me about your day." "My day was great. Molly took her first step. When she wakes up maybe we can get her to do it again." You get the picture. These conversations occur without much thought or concentration. We have thousands of casual conversations daily. They are usually pleasant and breezy. They begin quickly and end just as fast.

Although casual conversations are lighthearted, they often lack the emotional connection required for sexual desire. You have plenty of casual conversations, but few are sexual motivators.

The Informational Conversation

The main purpose of this type of conversation is the exchange of information. It is used to discuss the news events or politics of the day, your project at work, or your mother-in-law's medical exam. It's a conversation that involves any topic not involving your relationship. Just because you talk to each other about that vacation you are planning together doesn't mean you are communicating at all about your relationship. This type of conversation can be stimulating or boring as well. This, of course, depends on whether or not you're interested in the topic being discussed.

During an informational conversation, you may share your personal thoughts, feelings, and opinions, but there is no intention of either trying to get close or resolving a conflict. As in casual conversations, emotional intimacy is missing. Although you may express an emotion while discussing a newsworthy event, the emotion has little to do with your personal relationship.

Let's simplify these distinctions. If you are having a conversation with your partner and that conversation could easily be had with any other person on the planet, you are involved in either a casual or informational conversation. If you are having a conversation with your partner that could not be had with anyone else on the planet, you are involved in a connected conversation. Now, let's take a look at the most important conversation within your relationship, the connected conversation.

The Connected Conversation

A connected conversation is verbal intercourse that requires individual power, power reciprocity, effective communication, and conversational skills. This type of conversation is the seat of passion.

A connected conversation is an essential component to your sexual relationship. If you don't believe me, listen to the hundreds of women I've interviewed who rank the lack of connectedness as the number two reason for not wanting to be sexual with their partners. Remember, the number one reason is the powerlessness factor.

A connected conversation is filled with feeling messages, relating only to your relationship. During this conversation, nothing else matters. Not a discussion of world events, not a discussion of the children, not a discussion of what you did at work. Let's take a look at the essential and positive components needed in a connected conversation.

Self-Disclosure

You must be willing to share your most personal and intimate feelings with your partner and vice versa. If you are authentically revealing emotions but your partner is not, you are not engaging in a connected conversation.

Courage

Sharing personal and intimate information with your partner can trigger feelings of vulnerability. It takes courage to self-disclose. A rule of thumb is the more you share, the more intimate and connected you become to your partner.

Trust

While revealing feelings that are extremely personal in nature, you have to believe that your partner will respect and cherish your feelings, and your partner has to be reassured that you will do the same.

Unfortunately, however, personal information shared with your partner could possibly be used as artillery during a future argument. If this happens, it prevents the possibility of having another connected conversation again. A simple remedy would be to promise each other that you will respect and cherish any personal information shared today and always. Keep in mind that when you share your thoughts, feelings, and opinions, this is the most wonderful gift you can offer to one another.

Understanding

I've interviewed thousands of individuals who told me that feeling understood by their partner is fundamental to their happiness. I once interviewed a woman who burst out crying with tears of relief when I said, "I totally understand what you're saying." She was elated when she felt that the message she was trying to convey was understood. As mentioned, repeating back your partner's message will insure that your interpretation was correct.

Validation

When you and your partner have a difference of opinion, how do you deal with the disagreement? Do you tell your partner that they are wrong and you are right? Or, do you each affirm the other's point of view. You don't need to agree; however, you need to accept one another's viewpoint. Keep in mind that there are no wrong points of view, only different ones.

Interest

Have you ever observed two people who just met and are attracted to one another? They are totally interested in getting to know each other. They ask questions of each other and listen intently to the answers. After they think they know one another, however, this intentional interest goes down the tubes. It's as if there is nothing more to learn about each other. Of course this is untrue. Each and every day we change. Happily, I'm not the same woman that I was at twenty, thirty, forty, or fifty. My husband is not the same person as he was at twenty, and so forth. Hopefully, we continue to grow and learn until the day we die. Yet, many couples stop asking questions of interest regarding their partners. Why? People honestly believe, from the bottom of their hearts, that they truly know their partners just because they have been living together for a period of time. What a mistake! For example, female client told me recently that her partner was "not the man she married ten years ago." I should hope not! The problem was that she wasn't taking the time to get to know the man he was today. He, in turn, wasn't taking the time to share who he was with her.

When couples get bored with one another, it's because they really have failed to notice that their partner has changed. Once you become more interested, rather than trying to be interesting, the boredom will fly out of your relationship.

Here is one way to get to know your partner better. Each morning, while drinking your coffee, ask your partner one question about him or her. It can be about anything. You may be shocked to find out that your partner has totally changed regarding something that you thought you already knew about him or her. That's the exciting part of being in a relationship. Welcome change, embrace it, and share your changes with your partner.

Being Present in the Here and Now

While engaged in a connected conversation, were you concentrating on what was being discussed or were you thinking of something else? When you are present, nothing else matters but the conversation at hand. There is nothing more annoying than having a conversation with someone who is inattentive. You get the feeling that you are talking to a block of wood.

Equally annoying is the sidetracking of a connected conversation. Here, while in the midst of a conversation in the here and now, a totally different past issue is somehow dragged into it. That can only happen if either you or your partner is not present in the current conversation. When you are being present, you'll stick to the issue at hand and only discuss that. In other words, you can't be in the past or the future or anywhere else. You have to remain in the present.

Affection

Showing affection and having it returned enhances intimacy during a connected conversation. By touching and being touched, by kissing and being kissed, by embracing and being embraced, this will add a whole new dimension to verbal intercourse. I don't know of one single person who doesn't enjoy the wonderful and sensuous experience of being touched by someone they love. Demonstrative behavior is one of the most powerful ways to show love and enhance connection. During your connected conversation, hold hands. This enhances nonverbal power reciprocity.

Empathy

This skill, and it is a skill, is essential to a connected conversation. When you have the ability to put yourself in your partner's shoes, you will better understand what your partner is feeling about an issue and vice versa. I treated a couple where the woman was feeling upset because, during a social event, her husband danced with one particular woman most of the evening. He felt he did nothing wrong and could not understand why she was upset, until I said, "How would you feel if your wife danced with another man all night?" He looked as if I just punched him in the stomach. He said, "Oh, I see what you mean, I'd be more than upset, I'd be furious!" If both of you cannot understand one another's feelings, how can you resolve any type of conflict during a connected conversation?

Authenticity

During any conversation, you need to be totally yourself. I've watched couples say things to one another that weren't true to their feelings at all. Why would someone be phony? To look good, that's why. For example, a male client told me that he wasn't jealous or threatened when his wife went out to lunch with a very good-looking male coworker because he totally trusted his wife. I asked him what trusting his wife had to do with his feelings. He finally admitted that he was extremely jealous and quite threatened. Of course he was; if he loves his wife, picturing her with another sexy man would make any man feel jealous and threatened. I asked him why it took him so long to get in touch with his true feelings. He said, "I didn't want her to think I didn't trust her, but mostly I didn't want her to see my insecurities." As you can clearly see, he wanted to look like he was the most secure man on the planet; he was above looking insecure. There is nothing in the world more charming than an authentic person.

Now, let's take a look at the negative characteristics that can create disconnection during a conversation. If you take all of the positive characteristics described above and do the *opposite,* you'll have most of the negative characteristics. These create distance and have no place in a connected conversation. There are, however, three major negative characteristics that seem to stand out more than any others. Criticism, withdrawal, and mind reading are considered to be the most prominent characteristics that will bring a connected conversation to a screeching halt.

Criticism

Criticism occurs when one person finds fault with their partner and lets their partner know it verbally. Criticism is being judgmental. It's nit-picking. It's making your partner wrong. It's airing a complaint in an offensive and abusive manner. It's attacking the person rather than the person's behavior. It's ugly and it hurts my heart when I have to witness it. Criticism can take many forms. "Why were you so talkative during dinner? No one could get a word in edgewise." Or, "Why do you say things before thinking them through?" Or, "Must you eat so fast?" Or, "The way you drive makes me nervous." Or, "I can't believe you're going to wear that to a party."

I'm not saying that you should never air a complaint, because you should. Actually, there's nothing healthier. It's the only way to work on conflict. Here's the distinction between a complaint and a criticism. A complaint addresses the issue or behavior. A criticism attacks the person. For example, a complaint is, "I feel annoyed when you leave the toilet seat up." A criticism is, "You are annoying when you leave the toilet seat up." As you can see, the first example uses "I feel" at the beginning of the statement, by which the speaker assumes responsibility for the feeling of irritation. The second example uses "you" at the beginning of the statement, by which the speaker is placing blame and attacks the partner. This will create defensiveness in the listener. You certainly have the right to request that the toilet seat remain down so you don't fall in during the middle of the night. There is, however, a positive way to make this request. It's essential to remove criticism from your conversations.

Withdrawing and Shutting Down

There is nothing more annoying than watching a partner withdraw from a conversation. How do they do this? Easy, they just go somewhere else either mentally or physically. They disconnect from their partner or they leave the scene. Actually, I have been known to shut down during a conversation, especially when it's not going my way. Although I don't do this often, I have to work very hard on remaining present and not going away.

Why do individuals shut down or withdraw? Because they are threatened by the issue being discussed, or they are protecting themselves from being hurt, or they are bored by the conversation, or they haven't been taught how to share feelings authentically. You cannot have a connected conversation when only one person is present.

Mind Reading

Over time, we begin to think that we know our partner like a book. The truth is, we probably do in many situations. We most likely know what makes them happy, sad, or angry. The one thing, however, that none of us can do is read minds. Yet, we all do it on a daily basis. There is nothing more annoying than hearing our partner make statements like, "I know you don't feel attracted to me anymore because I've gained weight." The truth is that you yourself are feeling unattractive due to weight gain. Maybe your partner feels the same, maybe not. You have to ask, "Do you still find me attractive?" Unless something is said out loud, don't assume you know what your partner is thinking.

If you work at enhancing the positive components and eliminating the negative ones, your connected conversation will be powerful. Always keep in mind that, during a connected conversation, your words must be carefully chosen, and your message must be clear and succinct. This conversation always requires intense listening. You cannot be thinking of anything but what's being discussed at the moment. If your partner has lost sexual desire, I strongly suggest that you initiate a connected conversation for at least ten minutes a day to transform your relationship. Your partner will feel the intimate connection needed for sexual desire to be present.

The simple truth is, many couples never learned how to engage in a connected conversation. Connected conversations seem to be effortless for many women, but not for men. A good deal of the reason for this is that men and women are socialized differently. Women are taught to listen to what is said to them and encouraged to openly share their feelings. Men, on the other hand, are taught to speak, have others listen to them, and to keep their emotions (other than anger) in check. Thank goodness society is changing and we're finally encouraging our sons to be more expressive emotionally.

I am truly invested in getting men to totally understand how important connected conversations are to their relationship. Again, this should be an incentive; if your partner feels connected to you and there is power reciprocity, her sexual desire will increase. Have you ever heard your partner say something like this: "I can't turn myself on like a light switch when you want to make love. I need something to get me in the mood. I need to feel a connection to you."

What do you think she means by that? Does she mean that she needs you to get her chocolate or roses? Although it's a nice touch, that's not what she needs. Does she need you to warm her up by talking dirty? Nope, usually that's a turnoff for most women. What about telling her about that cute twenty-year-old that's recently been hired who came on to you? Definitely not.

Let me tell you about a couple who came to me for help; the woman's sexual desire was at an all-time low. Several attempts were made by her partner to get her in the mood. He simply didn't understand what she meant when she said that she needed to feel close to him before being sexual. He tried a romantic dinner, flowers, and candy. Nothing seemed to work.

Just before seeing this couple, he had finally thrown in the towel after his last effort. What was it? One evening, before climbing into bed, his wife mentioned that her nightgown looked like a rag. The next day, he remembered what she had said the night before and took time off from his busy schedule to shop for sexy lingerie. He could hardly wait to surprise his wife with this gift. He excitedly arrived home and handed her the gift without saying a word. What do you think she said after receiving her gift? "This isn't for me, it's for you! Do you think that if I slip this stupid-looking thing on, I'll magically turn into a sex goddess? Do you honestly think a nightgown is going to make me want to rush into the bedroom?" The poor guy was devastated. Although his intentions were admirable, this was not what she meant by getting close. If he engaged her in a connected conversation while she unwrapped the gift, the outcome could have been different. He might have said, "Honey, I remembered what you said about your nightgown, and I decided to buy you a new one. I hope you like it. If you don't, you can exchange it for something else."

Why do you think this would have made a difference? The gift would have validated the fact that he actually listened to her the night before when she said her nightgown was a rag. This definitely would have endeared him to her. The connection would have been that he honored her by listening to what she said the night before.

Exercise: Let's Connect

Connected conversations are rare among couples. For this reason, I'm going to ask you to practice having one right now. Are you ready?

- A key component is for you and your partner to be able to identify when a connected conversation begins. It takes practice. Let your partner know when you switch conversational styles. Similarly, check out with your partner when you think he or she has actually switched. With practice, you and your partner will be able to identify when the conversational style changes.

- When you would like to engage in a connected conversation, inform your partner at the start that you would like to switch into one. For example, "Robert, I'd like to switch to a connected conversation. Are you willing to switch?"

- When your partner agrees to have a connected conversation, begin the conversation by a self-disclosing statement. These statements usually begin with feeling words or phrases. For example, "I've been feeling ignored by you lately." Or, "I feel that we are drifting apart." Or, "I get the feeling that you are upset about something." Now, allow your partner to answer with a feeling response. For example, "Mary, I'm sorry that you feel as if I'm ignoring you; it makes me sad that you feel that way."

- Experience the safety and intimacy of your couple boundary and the use of effective communication skills. For example, I want you both to bring forth and feel that invisible circle that defines you as a couple. Stay in the moment—no mind reading—and remain on the topic. Most importantly, do not switch back into an informational or casual conversation. For example, note the switch to an informational conversation in the following. "Mary, I'm sorry that you feel ignored, but my boss has been putting so much pressure on me lately. I don't think I told you this, but our office is going through a downsizing process and the CEO is coming in next week to go over our books." Robert switched into an informational conversation when he began describing what happened rather than what he and Mary were feeling.

● Tap into your individual power and empower your partner.

Always reserve a connected conversation during times when you want to connect on an emotional and intimate level. You might find yourselves in an informational or casual conversation; however, if you or your partner would like to move into a connected conversation, you must be deliberate in your intention.

You've done great. Enjoy a connected conversation; the rewards are certainly well worth it. Now take a break and relax. The next and final chapter is designed to help ease you both into a connected conversation regarding your sex life.

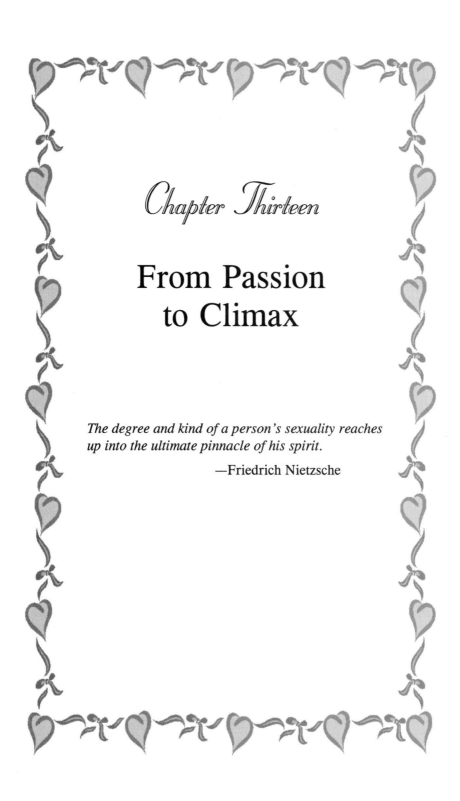

Chapter Thirteen

From Passion
to Climax

*The degree and kind of a person's sexuality reaches
up into the ultimate pinnacle of his spirit.*

—Friedrich Nietzsche

Despite the fact that you and your partner may consider yourselves to be sexually enlightened, you may still have a difficult time discussing sexual issues regarding your own sexual relationship. Sexuality is, and always has been, a difficult topic to discuss. Actually, I've not met too many couples who were comfortable sharing their sexual opinions, thoughts, and feelings with each other. Most couples, sexually savvy or not, would rather sweep the topic under the rug than have a connected sexual conversation.

Starting a Sexual Connected Conversation with Your Partner

Sex is a personal and private matter, as it should be. You must, however, be able to turn on your sex centers in order to avail yourself of that splendid possibility of turning your present sex life into something phenomenal. To accomplish this goal, you must engage in connected, sexual discussions with your partner. You have already acquired the skills of having powerful connected conversations. Now is the time to take these skills and integrate the topic of sex within your conversations.

There may, however, be two primary reasons stopping you from discussing sex. The first reason is the unpleasant feeling of shame that may accompany a frank sexual discussion. And, secondly, neither partner wants to hurt the other's feelings by stating that there may be something missing or something that needs to be changed in their sexual relationship.

There is no magic potion I can offer to break through this embarrassment. I can, however, offer a brief explanation. Most of us were raised in sexually repressed homes and given negative sexual messages, such as sex is dirty and shameful. In fact, most of us grew up never mentioning sex at all. It is imperative that you break through this embarrassment once and for all if you want to enrich your sex life.

Your initial sexual conversation with your partner during this next section may feel awkward and uncomfortable. I can promise you that the more you discuss sexual issues, the easier these conversations will become. This chapter contains sexually explicit information; sounds like the warning for X-rated material. I suppose, in some respects, it is. I am frequently struck by the fact that the media continues to push the envelope in an attempt to titillate its viewers. And viewers seem to need more and more sexually graphic content to become titillated. We have made the leap from *I Love Lucy* to *Sex and the City*. Yet, very few couples have made a similar leap in their sexual conversations with their partners. Most couples experience little or no embarrassment while watching a movie where nude couples go down on each other; they may have the thought, "Gee, that looks like a lot of fun." They may think it, but they rarely have the power to verbalize this to their partner. Instead, embarrassment prevents them from using a particular sexual scenario as an opportunity for discussion that could possibly enrich their sex lives. Embarrassment and the shame attached are the antithesis to a rewarding, fun, and enriched sex life. The following illustration speaks to the importance of engaging in sexual conversations.

Ann and Roger, both physicians at a local hospital, requested couple therapy because Roger was considering a divorce. Although their ten-year marriage was "mostly happy," their sex life was dismal. During the past two years, Ann was suffering from a sexual desire disorder. She had absolutely zero interest in sex. As a result, Roger felt unloved, angry, and confused. He mistakenly thought that if he romanced her by bringing her flowers, candy, and taking her to candlelit restaurants, she would magically be transformed into a sex goddess. When that proved to be unsuccessful, he felt thwarted, angry, and discouraged.

Roger began to berate Ann, stating that there was something "sexually wrong with her," and she should seek professional help to "fix her." Ann responded to his rebuke by accepting total responsibility for her lack of libido and sought counsel with a local therapist who was unfamiliar with the phase of sexual desire as explained in this book.

During the course of therapy, it was brought out that Ann had been faking orgasms throughout her marriage. After lovemaking, Ann would secretly masturbate herself to orgasm. Her therapist erroneously considered inorgasmia to be the primary problem. That, however, was not Ann's problem. Ann could have orgasms, but not with Roger. Her therapist then asked if Roger was an adequate lover. Ann responded, "Yes, he is a gentle lover and also performs cunnilingus." The therapist informed Ann that she may be holding back in an unconscious attempt to punish Roger for some past indiscretion. Ann couldn't think of any reason to punish Roger, and there were no past indiscretions. Then her therapist made a gentle inquiry that perhaps Ann was no longer in love with Roger. That wasn't it either; Ann loved Roger with all her heart.

Eventually, Ann dropped out of individual therapy, feeling hopeless and helpless. This well-intentioned therapist was attempting to treat the orgasm phase rather than the desire phase. As mentioned, if the diagnosis is incorrect, the treatment will be unsuccessful.

Roger confided in a colleague regarding his unhappy sex life. His friend knew that I was a sex therapist and was aware that I only treated couples, not individuals. Roger discussed this with Ann, and they both agreed to enter sex therapy as a couple.

I learned that they both were raised in strict religious families that considered any topic of sexuality taboo. And as adults, this attitude prevailed, preventing them from having intimate, sexual discussions. When I began to ask specific questions regarding their sex life, they blushed and looked as if I'd just asked them to strip naked. Keep in mind that they were physicians, yet like most people, they reacted with a great degree of embarrassment. I explained that the first ground rule of therapy is to persevere through the shame, because we will be having frank, honest, sexual discussions.

Ann and Roger's first task was to figure out when Ann's libido dropped, the possible obstacles interfering with her desire, and what Roger was doing or not doing to contribute to Ann's lack of motivation.

While discussing their assignment, it was clear that they were engaging in an informational conversation, one filled with facts and intellectual jargon. Neither of them possessed power since they could not state their personal opinions, thoughts, and feelings persuasively, making reciprocity impossible. Ann had not yet shared her secret, revealed to her former therapist, and Roger continued to believe that Ann's problem was her own psychological one.

During the next few weeks, I took them through the same process you and your partner have gone through in this book. They learned everything there was to know about their desire disorder. They were able to develop a healthy couple boundary. They learned effective communication skills and how to use them during a connected conversation. They were each able to tap into their power and empower each other. Now it was time to take a look at the cause of their desire disorder. Yes, it was time to talk about sex.

I had them face each other and answer the following questions, "Ann, do you adequately lubricate?" Her response was, "Yes." "Roger, are you able to achieve and maintain an erection during lovemaking?" He answered, "Yes." "Can you each achieve orgasm?" "Yes," they each answered. "Most of the time, do you experience orgasm during lovemaking?" Roger answered, "Yes," but Ann remained silent. Finally, after a long five minutes, Ann revealed her secret to Roger. She had been faking orgasms throughout their entire marriage. Roger was flabbergasted. He wanted to know why she had been faking all these years. She tearfully explained that it took her forever to climax, and she didn't want Roger to have to wait that long to enter her vagina. Unbeknownst to Roger, he wasn't taking the time required to bring Ann to orgasm. And Ann was too embarrassed to tell him.

As you can clearly see, Ann's issues had little to do with orgasm. She had a desire disorder based on the fact that she did not perceive lovemaking as being all that exciting and enjoyable. She perceived sex as being mostly penetration, with occasional oral sex thrown in. Let's face it, if you love chocolate, you will develop cravings for this delicious treat. If, however, you perceived chocolate as being sugarless and bitter, you would certainly not develop a craving. That's what happened to Ann. She perceived lovemaking as something uneventful.

Once Ann was able to explain to Roger that it took her at least forty-five minutes of clitoral stimulation to achieve orgasm, he happily agreed to give her all the time she needed. By the way, any amount of time is normal. Some women can have an orgasm in five minutes, and others take longer than Ann.

What may have looked like an orgasmic dysfunction was actually a sexual desire disorder. Nor was her disorder based on deep-rooted psychological problems or an earth-shattering obstacle. Once they openly and powerfully discussed sex, they were able to restore sexual desire.

I'm pleased to report that Ann is now enjoying orgasms during lovemaking, and Roger is quite happy to give Ann all the time she requires. In addition, they began to explore many other sexual likes and dislikes. The more they talked, the less embarrassment they felt.

As you can see from the above illustration, being able to have a powerful, connected conversation with your partner about sexuality increases sexual desire and enhances all sexual activities. Like Ann and Roger, you can't magically expect to have a great sex life if you can't even talk about sex. After all, your partner is your best friend with whom you should be able to share anything. So, start sharing.

Each and every one of us has different sexual needs and desires that we have to address verbally to our partner. Some of us would like to have sex daily. Some of us are satisfied with once a month. Some of us enjoy oral sex and some do not. Some like experimenting with new and creative sexual positions; some are satisfied with the missionary position. Some like long and luxurious foreplay and some like quickies. In addition, these sexual needs and desires change daily. You may enjoy oral sex on a Monday, but on Saturday it's the last thing you feel like doing. Each and every time is different. That's what makes sex so interesting. You have to continually let your partner in on your changing needs and desires. Don't make the same mistake that Ann and Roger made; a great sex life doesn't happen magically, it takes frank discussions.

Discussions Involving the Three Phases of the Sexual Response Cycle

In the introduction I briefly touched on the three phases of the human response cycle (Masters and Johnson 1966). Now I will provide you with a little more detail. The reason is to acquaint you with enough information to facilitate your own sexual discussions. In addition, I'd like to remind you that a sexual activity is not limited to intercourse. There are zillions of sexual activities that suit the taste of our own uniqueness. The more common sexual activities may include: oral sex, anal sex, taking showers together, masturbating in front of each other, sensual massage, sexual massage, tying each other up during foreplay, blindfolding each other during foreplay, viewing or reading erotic material, rubbing each others feet, embracing, kissing, lying naked on the beach, holding hands, washing each others' hair, acting out sexual fantasies, slathering each other with chocolate or whipped cream and slowly licking it off, just to name a few. A sexual activity is anything that you consider a turn-on and sexually enjoyable. Be creative and have fun with sex.

As I briefly discuss the three phases, I'd like you and your partner to answer questions at the end of each phase. These questions are designed to facilitate powerful, sexually connected conversations. Use your power and power reciprocity. These questions are only samples. You are welcome to make up your own. Have fun during these conversations!

Phase One: Desire

As you know by now, desire is the first phase of the human response cycle, where an individual longs for or strongly wants to seek out sexual expression. To maintain or recapture the highest level of sexual desire uniquely possible within your relationship, you must have a healthy couple boundary; possesses individual power; be able to exchange this power within a connected conversation; and be able to discuss sexual issues.

What Men Need to Know about Women during Desire

- As mentioned before, if her sex centers are not turned on in the kitchen, sex will be either ho-hum in the bedroom or there will be no sex at all. It is essential to engage in a powerful connected conversation.

- In my experience as a therapist, most women will seldom have as much sexual desire as men have. No one exactly knows the reason for this. An explanation could be that men produce more testosterone and the male brain has a larger hypothalamus. But who knows? The important thing is to not take this fact as rejection.

- Most women I've interviewed would love to touch, kiss, embrace, and massage their partners but refrain from doing so. Why? They are afraid that these intimate gestures will automatically be interpreted as a trigger for intercourse. If you engage her in connected conversation about this and guarantee her that you won't whisk her away to the bedroom, you'll enjoy the pleasures that these intimate gestures bring without necessarily leading to intercourse.

- Most women are embarrassed about their sexual fantasies. Encourage her to discuss them, and who knows, maybe you'll be role-playing one of her favorites.

- Tell her on a daily basis why you love being her life partner. I know most of you think it, but thinking is silent. You must verbally express it.

- Most women adore receiving love notes. Go ahead, leave a short one on her pillow before going off to work and see what happens. In addition, take a thirty-second break from your busy day and call to let her know you love her. That is also a turn-on.

- Don't even bother trying to get close to her sexually after a heated argument. Give her plenty of time and space to blow her anger off.

- Most women are tactile. Touching her is essential. Hold her hand, rub her neck, kiss her, and embrace her. Touching helps to turn on her sex centers.

- Candles, rose petals, love notes, soft music, and chocolate are nice touches, but that's not what will turn on her sex centers. It's the thought behind these romantic gestures that will. Keep in mind, individual power and power reciprocity is the only aphrodisiac that works. When you treat her lovingly, she will respond lovingly, and when she responds lovingly, fireworks will explode.

- Most women get more turned on watching a romantic love scene compared to graphic sex, including pornography.

- Although women are not as turned on visually as are men, they do, however, like those silk boxers or pajamas.

What Women Need to Know about Men during Desire

- If you are not already aware, men are turned on visually. Although the excitement generated by the models in Victoria's Secret's yearly TV program certainly speaks to this, the turn-on for men is imagining how their partner will look in this sexy attire. Plus, for some unknown reason, they love the color red. Go ahead, throw away those cotton gowns and buy some sexy stuff.

- Most men have a much greater motivation for sexual inter-course than most of you have. That's perfectly normal. Gently explain to them that there are a million other sexual activities to engage in, like a massage or hugging, before going to sleep.

- After a heated argument, most men have no problem request-ing sex. Don't get offended. They are fearful that the argument has distanced the two of you, and it's their way of getting close again.

- Most men love to engage in sexual fantasy. Go ahead, ask him if he would like to engage in one.

- Most men need to hear that they are valued, appreciated, and loved. Validate him on a daily basis. Men love to hear that you think how deliciously handsome they are.

- Most men will never fully comprehend that a connected conversation is paramount to your sexual desire. It is your responsibility to teach him just how important it is to your relationship. Let him know repeatedly that an intimate conversation is key to your sexual desire.

- Contrary to popular belief, many young men experience a temporary drop in libido. Also, as men age, they experience a fading of desire. This can profoundly affect their self-esteem. When this occurs, men feel vulnerable and embarrassed, fearful that they might have lost part of their identity forever. It takes a connected conversation to deal with these changes. Most often this drop is not permanent; your powerful connected conversations, along with the information in this book, can resolve his drop in libido.

- Most men lose their desire completely when their partner acts powerless or childlike. Remember the wimp factor, and turn on your power.

Titillating and Information Gathering Questions to Ask Each Other

- What are your favorite sexual fantasies? Please remember my word of warning; don't share fantasies that either exclude your partner or include someone you personally know, or are otherwise threatening.

- Would you like to act out these fantasies with one another? Men are turned on visually and enjoy it when their female partner dresses up sexy.

- Do you masturbate? If not, why? Masturbation is healthy and fun, even if you are having sex on a regular basis. It keeps vasocongestion (the rushing of blood to the genitals) and myotonia (muscle tension) in healthy working condition. Plus, it keeps those fantasies fresh and new.

- Do you like those romantic gestures that are an adjunct to desire? Candlelit dinner, soft music, fresh flowers, favorite fragrances, love notes, love gifts, and loving phone calls are always a lovely and welcome touch. Women seem to need romance more than men do.

- Do you stroke each other's ego? I can't stress enough how important it is to compliment one another's appearance. Go ahead; do you like your partner's eyes, hair, mouth, nose, voice, body? Letting your partner know you perceive their physical appearance as sexy goes a long way. Very few of us think that we are all that attractive. It's great to hear it from our partner. I always tell my husband how cute he looks before he leaves for work.

- How often do you engage in connected conversations? You should both connect at least once a day.

- Do you perceive one another as powerful? By now, I'm sure you do.

- Are you using your power reciprocity? What you give is what you get.

- Do you daydream about a previous exciting sexual experience you had with your partner? If so, that keeps your fantasy life alive. If not, create one tonight.

Phase Two: Arousal

This is the second phase of the human response cycle. During this phase, you and your partner will go through similar neurophysiologic changes. Breathing becomes heavy, heart rate and blood pressure will increase, a flushing of the skin occurs, visual and auditory acuity becomes diminished, nipples become erect, blood rushes to the genitals, and muscle tension will begin to occur.

For Women

The inner two-thirds of the vagina will expand, inner lips of the vulva change color and swell, the clitoris slowly becomes enlarged, and at the height of arousal, the clitoris is pulled up and under the clitoral hood, and lubrication is released through the vaginal wall. Lubrication is necessary because it makes clitoral stimulation and intercourse more pleasurable. Normal levels of estrogen are essential for natural lubrication. If, however, there are particular reasons why you are not able to naturally lubricate, you can use an over-the-counter lubricant, a non-irritating oil or lotion, or saliva as a replacement.

Unlike the penis, which has two functions (urination and sex), the clitoris has no other function than to give you pleasure.

For Men

The rush of blood causes the penis to become erect, the scrotum thickens, the testes increase in size, the head of the penis becomes slightly enlarged, and preejaculatory fluid may appear. Although this fluid is not semen, it does contain some sperm. Erection makes insertion of the penis into the vagina possible. Men become aroused much quicker than women.

What Men Need to Know about Women during Arousal

- It takes women a much longer time to lubricate than it takes men to have an erection. Don't rush into things. Women are aroused by tactile stimulation. They need kissing, hugging, stroking, having their nipples sucked, and every other creative thing you can think of. Take it slow; foreplay needs to be savored.

- Most women do not enjoy having their clitoris stimulated until it is totally lubricated. You can enhance lubrication by applying a lubricant or using your saliva.

- Enthusiastic or vigorous manual stimulation can be perceived as being too rough. The clitoris is exquisitely sensitive. Ask her the type of stimulation she enjoys.

- Direct clitoral stimulation can be so intense that it can be perceived as being unpleasant. You can move to areas around and above the clitoris. Some women, however, do prefer direct clitoral stimulation. Ask you partner what she prefers.

- Few women like the one-way approach. They prefer it when their partner moves away from the clitoris altogether and returns to it seconds later.

- Most men love performing cunnilingus on their partner. However, some women love it and some don't; check it out with her. If she is uncomfortable with this idea, use your power and reciprocity to see if at least she'd like to try it one time. Who knows? She may enjoy the experience. If she doesn't, you have to respect her wishes.

- If your partner does enjoy cunnilingus, treat the clitoris gently. You can use your tongue to stimulate or suck.

- Men have a tendency to focus on the clitoris and the clitoris only. However, most women love long, sumptuous kissing, tender embracing, having their breasts fondled and sucked, their butt grabbed, and their anus gently stroked. Be creative; there are hundreds of erogenous zones on her body. The best way to discover other erotic zones is to give her a nonsexual massage. Avoid her genitals and breasts and just enjoy the rest of her body. Most women adore this.

- Before engaging in any sexual activity, make sure you've taken a shower and brushed your teeth. Most couples don't want to hurt their partner's feelings by asking them to do this.

- Do not attempt penetration until your partner has had at least one orgasm. Women are multiorgasmic. The more orgasms she has prior to penile penetration, the more enjoyable intercourse will be.

- Based on my experience as a therapist, very few women actually experience orgasm during sex. Most often, a woman can have an orgasm manually or by oral clitoral stimulation. If, however, during penetration, the penis rubs against or pulls on the clitoris, then she will have an orgasm. Women do, however, enjoy the pressure of having the penis deep inside and the thrusting involved.

  A small minority of women state that they do experience orgasm and ejaculation during intercourse when their G spot

(Grafenberg 1950) is stimulated. This G spot is located on the front wall of the vagina. It's a small, pea-sized area of tissue located midway between the opening of the vagina and cervix. Research on the G spot continues to be controversial. But I encourage couples to be adventurous and experiment.

- Many women enjoy vigorous thrusting during intercourse, and others prefer a gentle, smooth approach. Ask her what she likes.

- Some women like talking during foreplay, and others hate it. Ask her.

- Every woman on the face of the planet loves to engage in sensual massage. It's an extremely erotic sexual activity. An erotic massage might exclude breast and genital touching or intercourse. But I can guarantee that this massage will arouse her more than you can imagine. Many women feel that their male partner is only interested in her clitoris, breasts, and vagina during lovemaking. Our skin is the largest sex organ on our body. Try pleasuring all this area and watch her arousal soar.

What Women Need to Know about Men during Arousal

- The average size of an erect penis is around five inches more or less. Men are just as sensitive about penis size as women are about breast size. Let him know that the size of his penis is just perfect.

- Many men require tactile or oral stimulation during this phase. As a man ages, he will require more vigorous stimulation. Ask him what he likes.

- If a man is in good physical health, he will naturally have an erection, given the right incentives.

- After the age of forty, the penis no longer gets as hard as it did in the past. After fifty, he no longer achieves erection by the mere sight or touch of his partner's body. Now he needs more rigorous stimulation from his partner. Sex, however, remains exciting and pleasurable throughout his lifetime.

- The most sensitive area of the penis is the glans, or head.

- The scrotum, the sack that contains the testicles, is extremely sensitive. Be careful that you don't become too enthusiastic and grab too vigorously.

- Most men love to have their perineum stroked. This is the area between the genitals and anus. Other erotically sensitive areas that give most men pleasure are his breasts, buttocks, anus (opening of the rectum), and the rectum itself by insertion of a finger. Ask him what he likes.

- Like women, most men have several erotic areas on their body. Men love massage; both sensual and sexual massage can be used to discover his erotic spots.

- Many men have the misguided idea that the longer they keep their erection during intercourse, the more enjoyment their female partner will experience. It is up to women to let men know that they do not need to have marathon sex.

- When a man focuses on his performance rather than getting lost in the sensual moment, it could cause him to develop performance anxiety. If this happens, he could experience difficulty getting and maintaining an erection.

- All men love fellatio. If you haven't tried it, give it a try. The penis feels like a smooth stick of satin in your mouth. To make it more appealing, you can apply chocolate, honey, or whipped cream and suck it off. If, however, this type of sexual activity is too adventurous, don't force yourself to do it. Never do anything that you don't want to.

Questions

- Are you able to achieve and maintain an erection?

- Are you satisfied with the amount of manual penile stimulation that your partner provides?

- Are you able to adequately lubricate?

- Are you satisfied with the amount of clitoral stimulation that your partner provides?

- Do you each enjoy oral sex? If so, move on to the next question.

- Would you like your partner to suck on your scrotum? Do you like sucking on your partner's scrotum?

- Would you like your partner to manually or orally stimulate your perineum?

- Would either of you like to play with each other's anus or insert your finger into each other's rectum? A warning to men: if you engage in any type of anal or rectal sexual activity, make sure that you wash thoroughly before inserting your finger or penis into her vagina.

- Does your partner suck on your breasts? Would you like him or her to spend more, less, or no time on this activity?

- Do you like your buttocks grabbed or massaged?

- Do you each enjoy an occasional quickie?

- Do you take enough time during foreplay to totally explore and enjoy one another's body?

- Does your partner use pleasurable pressure while stimulating your clitoris?

- Do you enjoy taking showers or baths by candlelight together?

- Do you like to talk during lovemaking?

- Do you like to talk "dirty" during lovemaking?

- Would you like to use props occasionally during lovemaking—such as chocolate sauce, whipped cream, grapes, a vibrator, or anything else you can conjure up?

- Do you need your partner to take a shower, brush their teeth, or wear a fragrance prior to engaging in a sexual activity?

- Does skinny-dipping sound like fun?

- Would you like to engage in a sensual massage that does not lead to intercourse?

- Would you like to experiment with more novel sexual activities—such as taking turns tying each other up, using a blindfold, and performing oral sex on each other.

- Do you enjoy anal penetration?

- Would you like your partner to masturbate in front of you?

- Would you like to occasionally partake in a sexual activity without it leading to intercourse?

Phase Three: Orgasm

This is the third phase of the response cycle. This phase is considered the most pleasurable of all sexual sensations. Men and women alike continue to go through neurophysiological changes. Heart rate, blood pressure, and respiratory rates peak. There is a loss of muscle control, and there may be spasms of certain muscle groups in the face, hands, feet, and genital area.

For Men

Men experience contractions of the prostate, seminal vesicles, rectum, urethra, and penis. Ejaculation occurs shortly after these contractions begin. Ejaculation occurs in two stages. The first stage is emission. During this phase, the male will experience ejaculatory inevitability. In other words, he couldn't prevent coming even if he wanted to. The second stage is expulsion. He will experience contractions of the urethra, prostate, and the muscles at the base of the penis. The initial contractions will be the most pleasurable. This is when the semen is forcefully spurted from the urethral opening.

For Women

Women experience contractions of the uterus and rectal muscle. A female can have several orgasms in rapid succession, if she chooses. Now, you might think that this phase must include sexual intercourse, but it doesn't. Masturbation is enjoyable as well. If, however, you both would like to have intercourse, this is the ideal phase to have it in.

Women have a muscle, referred to as the PC muscle, that encompasses the vagina. If you keep this muscle in good working condition by exercising, your orgasm will be more intense. It's referred to as the Kegel exercise. The following will assist you in strengthening this muscle.

Exercise for Women

Pretend that you have to urinate but for whatever reason you have to hold it. Hold it, come on, squeeze—and then release. Now, place your finger inside your vagina and hold it. Can you feel the PC muscle squeezing your finger? If not, keep doing the squeeze exercise until you do. Practice this Kegel exercise without your finger as many times during the day as you'd like. You can do it anywhere, because no one can observe you doing it. The more you do it, the more you'll strengthen the muscle, and the more intense your orgasm will be.

As mentioned, the G spot has been given much publicity. This was named after a German gynecologist who first described it, Ernest Grafenberg (1950). The G spot is reported to be a highly sensitive, small, pealike mass of tissue located about two inches inside the vaginal opening toward the belly button. Supposedly, when this area is sexually stimulated, it can send a woman into wild sexual excitement and even cause ejaculation. Research, however, hasn't really proved this to be a fact. Many women report that they definitely have this sensitive area and they do ejaculate. If you feel you have this G spot, enjoy. If you don't, I wouldn't worry; it's not characteristic of most women.

For women, every orgasm is different. On a Monday, you could experience one that will send you to the moon. On Saturday, it might be just a small blip. These blips are pleasurable as well. Enjoy both types.

What Men Need to Know about Women during Orgasm

- Most women are multiorgasmic.

- Most, but not all, women do not enjoy swallowing semen during your orgasm.

- Despite what is portrayed in the movies, most women are less inclined to engage in solitary masturbation than are men. Encourage her to masturbate. When she discovers what she needs to experience orgasm, she'll be able to transfer this information to you.

- During orgasm, there is a loss of bodily control that could include passing gas. Try to get her to see the humor in this natural occurrence.

- Some women enjoy quickies as an alternative to long foreplay. It's up to both of you to powerfully negotiate this prior to lovemaking.

- There is a misconception that most women like intercourse to continue for an extended period of time. Most women I've interviewed stated that they don't really enjoy a long period of thrusting. In movies, intercourse goes on and on and on because it's titillating to watch. The reality is that after a few minutes of thrusting, it feels unpleasant to most women. Of course, there are some women who enjoy a long period of time. It's up to you to ask her.

- Most women like to be held after orgasm. I know you're spent, but force yourself to take a few minutes to embrace her. She'll feel valued, respected, and loved.

What Women Need to Know about Men during Orgasm

- There will be times that your partner will climax as soon as he gets close to the opening of the vagina or shortly after he enters. This can be disappointing, not only to him but to you as well. As mentioned, there are two phases of ejaculation, emission and expulsion. During emission the semen and sperm are propelled into the urethral bulb, where it remains seconds before it is expulsed. During those few seconds, he can delay orgasm if he pays close attention to what's happening in his body and if he also stops whatever he's doing or stops whatever you're doing. If, however, those seconds pass and sexual activity is not stopped, he'll come. Premature ejaculation is pretty simple to treat. It only takes a couple of sessions with a sex therapist.

- Usually, a man can only have one orgasm during lovemaking.

- Unlike women, most men do not enjoy further touching after orgasm is achieved. They are totally sated. All a man wants to do is roll over and sleep. Don't take this as being something negative. All this means is that he is spent, totally relaxed, and free from stress. This should make you feel great knowing that he will get a good night's sleep. Don't take this as a personal affront or an indication that he doesn't love or respect you. It's nature taking its course.

Questions

- Are you achieving orgasm?

- Would you like to have an orgasm without it leading to intercourse?

- Would you like to watch your partner masturbate?

- Would you like to experiment with different sexual positions?

- Is your favorite position with the man on top?

- Is menstruation a turnoff? If so, who is turned off?

- Do you like vigorous thrusting, or do you like the gentler approach?

- Is there anything missing from your current lovemaking? If so, what is it?

These, of course, are but a few questions to ask one another. Be tenacious while exploring your unique sexual preferences. And always keep in mind that, without desire, the above activities will lack intensity.

The Climax

I am certain that after reading this book and doing the exercises, you and your partner have successfully increased sexual desire. Any committed and loving relationship does, and always will, take work. I commend you and your partner for taking the time and energy that were required in completing this work. That certainly speaks to the importance of your cherished relationship.

I do, however, want you to keep in mind that sexual desire is rather ephemeral. It comes and goes at the drop of a hat. When desire is present, express your love. When it's not, reread the chapter on power and power reciprocity.

If, for any reason, you feel that you need more help than this book has provided, seek out the counsel of a sex therapist. Most are highly trained and may even hold an advanced degree in human sexuality. Sex therapists are extremely comfortable discussing sexual issues and understand that couples are initially embarrassed about discussing sexual matters. A sex therapist wants nothing more than to offer you and your partner treatment so that both of you will enjoy a more intimate, loving, and passionate relationship.

Thank you for letting me into your life. I feel honored that you have allowed me to be temporarily part of your relationship. Now that you have reached the end of this book, you and your partner are ready for a new and exciting phase in your commitment to each other. Visit my Web site at www.drcervenka.com for updated research, as well as upcoming media appearances and seminars.

References

Aponte, H.J., and J.M. Van Deusen. 1981. Structural family therapy. In *Handbook of Family Therapy,* edited by A.S. Gurman and Neil S. Jacobson. New York: Brunner Mazel.

Bateson, G. 1979. *Mind and Nature: A Necessary Unity.* New York: E.P. Dutton.

———. 1978. The birth of a double bind. In *Beyond the Double Bind,* edited by M. Berger. New York: Brunner Mazel.

———. 1958. *Naven.* Stanford, Calif.: Stanford University Press.

Bateson, G., and M.C. Bateson. 1972. *Steps to an Ecology of Mind: Collected Essays in Anthropology, Psychiatry, Evolution, and Epistemology.* Chicago: University of Chicago Press.

Beck, A.T. 1999. *Prisoners of Hate: The Cognitive Basis of Anger, Hostility, and Violence.* New York: HarperCollins.

———. 1989. *Love Is Never Enough.* New York: HarperCollins.

———. 1979a. *Anxiety Disorders and Phobias: A Cognitive Perspective.* New York: N A L.

———. 1979b. *Cognitive Therapy of Depression.* New York: Gulliver Books

———. 1976. *Cognitive Therapy and the Emotional Disorders.* New York: International Universities Press.

Carstensen, L.L., J.M. Gottman, and R.W. Levenson. 1995. Emotional behavior in long-term marriage. *Psychology and Aging* 10:140–49.

Cervenka, K.A., C.H. Brown, and R. Dembo. 1995. A family empowerment intervention of juvenile offenders. *Review of Aggression and Violent Behavior* 1: 205–16.

Dell, P. 1981. Beyond homeostasis. In *Foundations of Family Therapy,* edited by L. Hoffman. New York: Basic Books.

Donnelly, D. 1993. Sexually inactive marriages. *Journal of Sex Research* 30:171–79.

Gottman, J.M., and J. DeClaire. 2001. *The Relationship Cure: A Five-Step Guide to Building Better Connections with Family, Friends, and Lovers*. New York: Crown Publishers.

Gottman, J.M., and N. Silver. 1995. *Why Marriages Succeed or Fail: And How You Can Make Yours Last*. New York: Fireside.

Grafenberg, E. 1950. The role of urethra in female orgasm. *International Journal of Sexology* 3:145–48.

Hoffman, L. 1981. *Foundations of Family Therapy*. New York: Basic Books.

Kaplan, H.S. 1995. *The Sexual Desire Disorders: Dysfunctional Regulation of Sexual Motivation*. New York: Brunner Mazel.

———. 1974. *The New Sex Therapy: Active Treatment of Sexual Dysfunctions*. New York: Brunner Mazel.

Kinsey, A.C., W.B. Pomeroy, and C.E. Martin. 1953. *Sexual Behavior in the Human Female*. Philadelphia: W.B. Saunders.

———. 1948. *Sexual Behavior in the Human Male*. Philadelphia: W.B. Saunders.

Laumann, E.O., and R.T. Michael. 2001. *Sex, Love, and Health in America: Private Choices and Public Policies*. Chicago: The University of Chicago Press.

Lazarus, A.A. 1995. A multimodal perspective on problems of sexual desire. In *Sexual Desire Disorders,* edited by H.S. Kaplan. New York: Brunner Mazel.

Leiblum S.R., and R.C. Rosen. 1988. Introduction: Changing perspectives on sexual desire. In *Sexual Desire Disorders,* edited by S.R. Leiblum and R.C. Rosen. New York: Guliford Press.

LeVay, S. 1991. A difference in hypothalamic structure between heterosexual and homosexual men. *Science* 253:1034–1037.

———.1994. *The Sexual Brain*. Cambridge, Mass.: MIT Press.

Levenson, R.W., L.L. Carstensen, and J.M. Gottman. 1993. Long-term marriage: Age, gender, and satisfaction. *Psychology and Aging* 8:301–13.

Lief, H.I. 1985. Evaluation of inhibited sexual desire: Relationship aspects. In *Comprehensive Evaluation of Disorders of Sexual Desire,* edited by H.S. Kaplan. Washington, D.C.: American Psychiatric Press.

LoPiccolo, J., and J.M. Friedman. 1988. Broad-spectrum treatment of low sexual desire: Integration of cognitive, behavioral, and systemic therapy. In *Sexual Desire Disorders*, edited by S.R. Leiblum and R.C. Rosen. New York: Guliford Press.

Masters, W., and V. Johnson. 1966. *Human Sexual Response*. Boston: Little Brown.

Masters, W., V. Johnson, and R.C. Kolodny. 1994. *Heterosexuality*. New York: HarperPerennial.

Minuchin, S. 1981. *Family Therapy Techniques*. Cambridge, Mass.: Harvard University Press.

Minuchin, S., and M.P. Nichols. 1993. *Family Healing*. New York: Macmillan, Inc.

Money, J. 1994. *Reinterpreting the Unspeakable: Human Sexuality 2000*. New York: Continuum.

————. 1980. *Love and Love Sickness: The Science of Sex, Gender Differences, and Pair Bonding*. Baltimore, Md.: Johns Hopkins University Press.

Mulligan, T., and C.R. Moss. 1991. Sexuality and aging in male veterans: A cross-sectional study of interest, ability, and activity. *Archives of Sexual Behavior* 20:17-25.

Nichols, M.P. 1984. *Family Therapy Concepts and Methods*. New York: Gardner Press.

Ratey, J.J. 2002. *A User's Guide to the Brain*. New York: Vintage Books.

Schwartz, M., and W.H. Masters. 1988. Inhibited sexual desire: The Masters and Johnson Institute treatment model. In *Sexual Desire Disorders*, edited by S.R. Leiblum and R.C. Rosen. New York: Guliford Press.

Sternberg, R. 1986. A triangular theory of love. *Psychological Review* 93:119–35.

Tannen, D. 1990. *You Just Don't Understand: Women and Men in Conversation*. New York: Ballantine.

Trudel G., S. Aubin, and B. Matte. 1995. Sexual behaviors and pleasure in couples with hypoactive sexual desire. *Journal of Sex Education and Therapy* 21:210–16.

Westheimer, R. 1988. *Dr. Ruth's Guide to Good Sex*. New York: Simon & Schuster.

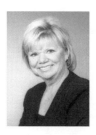 **Kathleen A. Cervenka, Ph.D.,** is a psychotherapist who holds a doctorate in human sexuality. She has been working for more than twenty years with couples on relationship issues and sexual dysfunctions. She provides sexual training seminars to professionals and makes frequent appearances on TV and radio. She lives in Belleair Beach, Florida with her husband.

Visit her at www.drcervenka.com

Some Other
New Harbinger Titles

The Stepparent's Survival Guide, Item SSG $17.95

Drugs and Your Kid, Item DYK $15.95

The Daughter-In-Law's Survival Guide, Item DSG $12.95

Whose Life Is It Anyway?, Item WLALW $14.95

It Happened to Me, Item IHPM $17.95

Act it Out, Item AIO $19.95

Parenting Your Older Adopted Child, Item PYAO $16.95

Boy Talk, Item BTLK $14.95

Talking to Alzheimer's, Item TTA $12.95

Helping a Child with Nonverbal Learning Disorder or Asperger's Syndrome, Item HCNL $14.95

The 50 Best Ways to Simplify Your Life, Item FWSL $11.95

When Anger Hurts Your Relationship, Item WARY $13.95

The Couple's Survival Workbook, Item CPSU $18.95

Loving Your Teenage Daughter, Item LYTD $14.95

The Hidden Feeling of Motherhood, Item HFM $14.95

Parenting Well When You're Depressed, Item PWWY $17.95

Thinking Pregnant, Item TKPG $13.95

Pregnancy Stories, Item PS $14.95

The Co-Parenting Survival Guide, Item CPSG $14.95

Family Guide to Emotional Wellness, Item FGEW $24.95

How to Survive and Thrive in an Empty Nest, Item NEST $13.95

Children of the Self-Absorbed, Item CSAB $14.95

The Adoption Reunion Survival Guide, Item ARSG $13.95

Call **toll free, 1-800-748-6273,** or log on to our online bookstore at **www.newharbinger.com** to order. Have your Visa or Mastercard number ready. Or send a check for the titles you want to New Harbinger Publications, Inc., 5674 Shattuck Ave., Oakland, CA 94609. Include $4.50 for the first book and 75¢ for each additional book, to cover shipping and handling. (California residents please include appropriate sales tax.) Allow two to five weeks for delivery.

Prices subject to change without notice.